WHAT THE DRUG COMPANIES WON'T TELL YOU

———— *and* ————

YOUR DOCTOR DOESN'T KNOW

WHAT THE
DRUG COMPANIES
WON'T TELL YOU

— *and* —

YOUR DOCTOR
DOESN'T KNOW

The Alternative Treatments That May
Change Your Life—And the Prescriptions
That Could Harm You

MICHAEL T. MURRAY, N.D.

ATRIA PAPERBACKS
New York   London   Toronto   Sydney

This publication contains the opinions and ideas of its author. It is intended to provide helpful and informative material on the subjects addressed in the publication. It is sold with the understanding that the author and publisher are not engaged in rendering medical, health, or any other kind of personal professional services in the book. The reader should consult his or her medical, health, or other competent professional before adopting any of the suggestions in this book or drawing inferences from it.

The author and publisher specifically disclaim all responsibility for any liability, loss, or risk, personal or otherwise, which is incurred as a consequence, directly or indirectly, of the use and application of any of the contents of this book.

ATRIA PAPERBACKS
A Division of Simon & Schuster, Inc.
1230 Avenue of the Americas
New York, NY 10020

Copyright © 2009 by Michael T. Murray, N.D.

First Atria Paperbacks edition May 2010

ATRIA PAPERBACKS and colophon are trademarks of Simon & Schuster, Inc.

For information about special discounts for bulk purchases, please contact Simon & Schuster Special Sales at 1-866-506-1949 or business@simonandschuster.com.

Designed by Jason Snyder

Manufactured in the United States of America

10 9 8 7 6 5

The Library of Congress has cataloged the hardcover edition as follows:

Murray, Michael T.
    What the drug companies won't tell you and your doctor doesn't know / Michael T. Murray.
        p.   cm.
    Includes bibliographical references and index.
    1. Naturopathy.   2. Alternative medicine.   3. Pharmaceutical industry—Corrupt practices—United States.   I. Title.
    RZ440.M88   2009
    615.5'35—dc22   2008019980

ISBN 978-1-4165-4933-8
ISBN 978-1-4165-4939-0 (pbk)
ISBN 978-1-4391-6429-7 (ebook)

In loving memory of my father, Clifford G. Murray, Jr.

ACKNOWLEDGMENTS

MOST OF ALL, I would like to acknowledge my wife, Gina. Her love, support, and patience are the major blessings in my life along with our wonderful children, Alexa, Zachary, and our littlest angel, Addison.

I have also been blessed with many exceptional people whom I am very fortunate to be able to call my dear friends. In particular, I want to acknowledge the tremendous positive influence that Dr. Gaetano Morello has had on my life, as well as his generous assistance in helping me mold this book into its final form. Thank you, Gaetano. Others who deserve special mention for helping me conceptualize this book are Roland Gahler and everyone at Natural Factors, Dr. Joseph Pizzorno, and Dr. Michael Lyon. Thanks to you all.

Lastly, I am indebted to the team at Atria led by Judith Curr for all of their hard work in making this book as reader-friendly and practical as possible.

CONTENTS

APPENDIXES

PROLOGUE

"The enemy of the conventional wisdom is
not ideas but the march of events."
—John Kenneth Galbraith

THE TERM "CONVENTIONAL WISDOM" was coined by the noted economist John Kenneth Galbraith in his book *The Affluent Society*, in 1958. According to Galbraith, conventional wisdom is established if it is simple, convenient, comfortable, and comforting—though not necessarily true. Galbraith also said, "We associate truth with convenience, with what most closely accords with self-interest or personal well-being." People want to believe conventional wisdom because it is indeed so simple, convenient, comfortable and comforting, even if it may not be true. And once conventional wisdom on any topic is accepted, it becomes difficult to prove otherwise.

In the United States, the medical establishment has created the conventional wisdom that drug-oriented medicine is the best form of medicine. Yet many of these drugs only make us feel better in the short term, while exposing us to the risk of dependency, producing side effects worse than the condition being treated, or actually causing the condition to worsen. These substantial risks, and the rising costs associated with a drug-oriented medical system, are creating an opportunity for change.

Change is definitely coming; in fact, we are in the midst of it. There has been a subtle revolution in medicine for years, and a new paradigm is emerging. A paradigm is a model used to explain events. As our understanding of the environment and the human body evolves, new paradigms—new explanations—are developed. For example, in physics the cause-and-effect explanations of Descartes and Newton were superseded by quantum mechanics, Einstein's theory of relativity, and theoretical physics, which takes into consideration the tremendous interconnectedness of the universe.

The new paradigm in medicine also focuses on interconnectedness: in this case, of body, mind, emotions, social factors, and the environment in determining the status of an individual's health. And whereas the old paradigm viewed the body basically as a machine that can be fixed best with drugs and surgery, in the new, emerging model these measures are secondary to natural, noninvasive, techniques to promote health and healing. The relationship between the physician and the patient is also evolving. The era of the physician as a demigod is over. The era of self-empowerment is beginning.

NATUROPATHIC MEDICINE

By definition and philosophy most conventional medical doctors (M.D.s) practice allopathic medicine—the system of medicine that focuses primarily on treating disease rather than promoting health. In contrast, you may have noticed the N.D. after my name on the cover. This signifies that I am a naturopathic doctor. I graduated from Bastyr University with a doctorate in naturopathic medicine—a system that emphasizes prevention, treatment, and the promotion of optimal health through the use of natural, nontoxic therapies. The scope of practice of an N.D. includes all aspects of family and primary care, from pediatrics to geriatrics, as well as the full range of human health conditions including cancer. Naturopathic medicine is based on seven time-tested principles:

1. **First, do no harm.** N.D.s seek to do no harm with medical treatment; therefore, they employ safe and effective natural therapies.

2. **Employ the healing power of nature.** N.D.s believe that the body has considerable power to heal itself. The role of the physician is to facilitate and enhance this process with the aid of natural, nontoxic therapies.

3. **Identify and treat the cause.** N.D.s are trained to seek the underlying causes of a disease rather than simply suppress the symptoms. Symptoms are viewed as expressions of the body's attempt to heal,

whereas causes can spring from physical, mental-emotional, and spiritual levels.

4. **Treat the whole person.** N.D.s are trained to view an individual as a whole, composed of a complex set of physical, mental-emotional, spiritual, social, and other factors.

5. **The physician is a teacher.** The word "doctor" comes from the Latin *docere*, which means "to teach." N.D.s view our roles as primarily those of teachers: to educate, empower, and inspire our patients to assume more personal responsibility for their health by adopting a positive attitude, lifestyle, and diet.

6. **Prevention is the best cure.** N.D.s believe that an ounce of prevention is worth much more than a pound of cure. With regard to cancer, this saying is especially true. We are specialists in preventive medicine. Real prevention of death caused by cancer is achieved not only by early diagnosis, but also through education and encouraging life habits that support health.

7. **Establish health and wellness.** Our primary goals for our patients are to establish and maintain optimum health and to promote wellness. "Health" is defined as the state of optimal physical, mental, emotional, and spiritual well-being; "wellness" is defined as a state of health, characterized by a positive emotional state. Naturopathic physicians strive to increase the patient's level of wellness, regardless of the level of health or disease. Even in cases of severe disease such as cancer, a high level of wellness can often be achieved.

THE NEED FOR RATIONAL MEDICINE

When people refer to me as an expert in alternative medicine, I usually correct them. I am a proponent of what I like to describe as *rational* medicine, which combines the best of both conventional medicine and alternative methods. In fact, I believe a system is evolving and emerging that incorporates the best of both conventional medicine and what is currently labeled "alternative" medicine. My goal is to speed up this process. Just as we now view the conventional treatments in vogue at the beginning of the nineteenth century (e.g., mercury, bloodletting, and purges) as having been irrational, counterproductive, and in many cases harmful, so too will many of today's conventional treatments be judged in a similar light by the medical circles of tomorrow. However, there are many conventional medical practices and drugs that are completely rational. In fact, it would be irrational not to take advantage of modern medicine when appropriate. That said, there is no question that the majority of health complaints for which patients see doctors originate with dietary and lifestyle factors. Trying to treat the symptoms with a drug (a biochemical Band-Aid) often fails to address the underlying cause and as a result leads to side effects. Clearly, a more rational and truthful approach to health care is needed.

SOME WORDS OF CAUTION

Although this book discusses numerous natural medicines and approaches, it is not intended as a substitute for appropriate medical care. Please keep the following in mind as you read:

▸ Do not self-diagnose. Proper medical care is critical to good health. If you have concerns about any subject discussed in this book, please consult a physician, preferably a naturopathic doctor (N.D.), a nutritionally oriented medical doctor (M.D.) or doctor of osteopathy (D.O.), or some other specialist in natural health care.

▸ Make your physician aware of all the nutritional supplements or herbal products you are currently taking, to avoid possible negative interactions with any drugs you take.

▸ If you are currently taking prescription medications, you absolutely must work with your doctor before discontinuing any drug or altering any drug regimen.

▸ Most health conditions require a multifactorial solution: medical, nutritional, and lifestyle changes. Do not rely solely on a single area of focus. You can't just take pills and not change your diet, or follow a diet and take pills but ignore lifestyle issues. Any truly effective approach to health must be truly integrated.

MY HOPE

It is my sincere hope that you—and those you care about—will use the information provided in the following pages to achieve greater health and happiness. I also hope that you can all become advocates of change. The nineteenth-century philosopher Arthur Schopenhauer observed that truth passes through three phases: first, it is ridiculed; second, it is fiercely and violently opposed; and third, it becomes self-evident. However, this three-part progression does not happen automatically or magically. As Dr. Martin Luther King, Jr., said, duration is not enough: the mere passage of time does not create change. It requires ordinary people envisioning, acting and constructing the future. Each of us can help bring this progression into being—in part, by being "phase three" people currently living in a "phase one" and "phase two" world.

Live in good health with passion and joy!

Michael T. Murray, N.D.

1

A MATTER OF TRUST— MAKING MEDICINE OR MAKING MONEY?

*"Where large sums of money are concerned,
it is advisable to trust nobody."*
—Agatha Christie

IS IT REALLY POSSIBLE that American baby boomers and younger generations have been led down a road to poor health by the pharmaceutical industry and conventional medical practice? Have the very industries, organizations, and medical doctors responsible for designing our health care system created the catastrophe of skyrocketing medical costs? Are the drug companies so powerful that they exert virtually complete control over the Food and Drug Administration (FDA), medical schools, prestigious medical journals, and continuing medical education for physicians? Is it true that adverse reactions to over-the-counter (OTC) and prescription drugs are estimated to kill over 100,000 Americans a year, making these reactions the fourth-largest cause of death in the United States, behind cancer, heart disease, and strokes?

The answer to all these questions is yes. The pharmaceutical industry and the medical monopoly have created a health care crisis in America. In this book, we will, together, take a peek behind the curtain to expose some of the fallacies and shortcomings of many popular medications. It is absolutely true that most of us have been helped in almost magical ways by the wonders of modern medicine, but the reality is that conventional medicine has also created a lack of personal accountability and a complete reliance on little pills to cure what ails us. We now have on our hands a modern epidemic, consisting not only of diseases that are clearly a result of diet and lifestyle, but also of diseases due to the side effects of drugs used in their treatment.

The United States has by far the highest per capita use of conventional medicines and uses over more than 40 percent of all of the drugs produced in the world each year, according to the World Health Organization (WHO); but we are only forty-second in terms of life expectancy. We are definitely not getting our money's worth from our medicine. It is easy to demonize the greedy pharmaceutical industry, but the problem is much deeper than that. It is also easy to say that most medical doctors have simply been unknowing pawns in the drug companies' game of profits, never realizing that they have been led to perpetuate lies, half-truths, and incomplete science; but the reality is that the medical profession has done a questionable job in protecting the health of the patient. In fact, many doctors are willing players in the game. They do not mind. It represents easy money. The average income for a medical doctor is more than $200,000 per year, and many specialists, such as radiologists and heart surgeons, have an average income of more than $300,000 per year. It could be that there is one very big reason why many medical doctors do not practice preventive medicine—money. The average yearly income for a member of the American College of Preventive Medicine, a group of preventive medical doctors, is $100,000—a good income, but considerably less than half the average income for other medical specialties.

Also, it is estimated that drug companies spend more than $57.5 billion a year marketing to physicians. This figure includes about $14 billion for what is referred to in the industry as "unmonitored promotion"; it can include lavish vacations and getaways, ostensibly continuing medical education. With about 700,000 practicing physicians in the United States, it is estimated that the drug industry spends about $60,000 in marketing per physician.[1]

Do the Drug Companies Spend More on Marketing or Research?

According to a very detailed analysis by two Canadian researchers, Marc-André Gagnon and Joel Lexchin, "The Cost of Pushing Pills: A New Estimate of Pharmaceutical Promotion Expenditures in the United States,"[1] drug companies spend twice as much money on marketing as on research and development. Now, the U.S. General Accountability Office (GAO) says otherwise. Why the discrepancy? Well, it turns out that the data supplied to the GAO are from IMS, a firm specializing in pharmaceutical market intelligence. There are many concerns about the accuracy of the IMS data, chief among them being that the data are derived by asking the drug companies to supply them. The bottom line is that the IMS data are simply not consistent with other published sources, including data provided by the U.S. Office of Technology Assessment as well as information gathered from year-end financial reports from the drug companies themselves.[2]

DRUG COMPANIES, PROFITS, AND THE FDA

If anyone knows the depth of the deceit and false promises heaped on Americans by drug companies, it is Marcia Angell, M.D., former editor in chief of the *New England Journal of Medicine*, one of the most respected medical journals in the world. According to Dr. Angell, the pharmaceutical industry "has moved very far from its original high purpose of discovering and producing useful new drugs. Now primarily a marketing machine to sell drugs of dubious benefit, this industry uses its wealth and power to co-opt every institution that might stand in its way, including the U.S. Congress, the Food and Drug Administration, academic medical centers, and the medical profession itself."[3]

There is now considerable evidence that the drug companies exert significant control over the FDA and the drug approval process. More than half of the experts hired to advise the FDA on the safety and effectiveness of drugs have financial relationships with drug companies that will be helped or hurt by their decisions. Federal law generally prohibits the FDA from using experts with financial conflicts of interest, but the FDA waived this rule 800 times in a 15-month period from January 1998 to June 2000. In an analysis of all advisory panel meetings from 2001 to 2004, at least one member had a financial link to the drug's maker or a competitor in 73 percent of the meetings.[1, 2] The potential damage from such ties was exemplified in 2005, when the FDA convened a meeting to discuss the toxicity of the COX-2 inhibitors Vioxx, Celebrex, and Bextra. Had the ten committee members with ties to industry been precluded from voting, the committee would have voted against continued marketing for Vioxx and Bextra; instead, all three drugs received favorable votes.[3, 4] As a result these potentially dangerous drugs were allowed to stay on the market. That trend has created a huge problem, because 20 percent of all approved drugs over the last 25 years were later found to have serious side effects leading either to the withdrawal of the drug from market or to warning labels noting these serious side effects. The drug companies could afford to take a gamble on drugs like Vioxx, Celebrex, Avandia, OxyContin, and others because of the huge profits they could generate.

Since the 1950s, drugs have been the most profitable industry in America. In December 1959, the last year of the Eisenhower administration, the Senate Subcommittee on Antitrust and Monopoly reported on a yearlong investigation of the drug industry with the declaration that the public was not only being overcharged for drugs but was being ripped off for useless and sometimes harmful medicines. Three charges were leveled at the drug industry by the subcommittee: (1) Patents sustained predatory prices and excessive margins. (2) Costs and prices were extravagantly increased in order to fund marketing expenditures. (3) Most of the industry's new products were no more effective than lower-priced, established drugs on the market. Back in the 1950s, this report changed the image of drug companies: the companies had been seen as employing lifesaving "researchers in white coats" but were now seen as employing primarily zealous "sales reps in cars."

Has the situation changed in the last 50 years? Yes: it has gotten much better for the drug companies, at the public's expense. During the past 50 years drug costs have skyrocketed at a rate five times inflation. In 1960, the drug industry had a profit margin of 10.6 percent of sales. By 1992, this had increased to 13 percent. In 2005, it was 18 percent. Pfizer, the world's number one drug company, had a profit margin of 26 percent of sales.

In 1980, the average prescription cost $6.52; in 1992 the cost was $22.50; in 2006 it was $50.17. Drug costs are higher in the United States than anywhere else in the world. Most major industrial nations apply profit control to limit how much a drug company can charge for a drug. Because most drug companies market the same drug throughout the world, they rely on the United States for the bulk of their profits. In the United States, drug companies can increase the price of drugs without fear, because there is very little competition. In fact, there is more cooperation between drug companies to keep prices high than there is price competitiveness.[3, 4]

HIGHER-PRICED DRUGS + MORE PRESCRIPTIONS WRITTEN = HUGE PROFITS FOR DRUG COMPANIES

The simple sum expressed above is astronomical in real life because more people than ever before are being placed on high-priced drugs. For example, roughly 4 billion prescriptions were filled last year, about 12 prescriptions for every person in the United States. Are all these prescriptions necessary? Remember that the United States uses more than 40 percent of all the drugs in the world but ranks only forty-second in life expectancy; also, it ranks only thirty-seventh in the quality of its health system, according to WHO. The high cost of drugs is bankrupting our elderly population, and our society. The number of seniors who depend on prescription drugs is unbearable. In 1992, the average senior received 19.6 prescriptions per year; in 2005, that number had nearly doubled, to 34.4. The average person over the age of 55 is on eight or more prescription drugs at any one time.

According to a study by Fidelity Investment released in March 2006, a 65-year-old couple retiring today will need, on average, $200,000 set aside to pay for medical costs during retirement. A big chunk of that $200,000 will go to pay for expensive drugs that produce questionable results and raise considerable safety issues. For example, the current treatment of type 2 diabetes is very absurd. Now an American epidemic, diabetes is also a source of huge profits for drug companies, yet the research findings are quite clear—oral medications to treat type 2 diabetes do not alter the long-term development of the disease. Although the drugs are quite effective in the short term, they create a false sense of security: they ultimately fail and are then prescribed at higher dosages or in combination with other drugs, leading to increased mortality. That is right; the long-term use of these drugs is actually associated with an earlier death, compared with mortality in control groups of diabetics who are not given the drugs. Here are some additional facts:

▸ It is estimated that 70 percent of patients with chronic daily headaches suffer from drug-induced headaches.

▸ Sleeping pills interfere with normal sleep cycles, produce numerous side effects, and are addictive.

▸ Aspirin, ibuprofen, and other nonsteroidal drugs (NSAIDs) used for arthritis lead to joint destruction by inhibiting the formation of cartilage.

▸ NSAIDs cause 16,500 deaths in the United States annually, and more than 100,000 Americans are hospitalized because of side effects.

▸ Acetaminophen overdose is the leading cause of acute liver failure and causes 10 percent of all cases of kidney failure.

▸ Drugs like Paxil, Zoloft, and Prozac contribute to obesity, but weight gain is not listed as a common side effect of these drugs.

WHY HAVE HEALTH CARE COSTS SKYROCKETED?

In addition to higher-priced drugs, the reasons often cited to explain the tremendous rise in health care costs include these:

Why Was the FDA Slow to Warn Patients about the Popular Diabetes Medication Avandia?

GlaxoSmithKline (GSK), the makers of the popular diabetes drug Avandia (rosiglitazone maleate) informed the FDA as early as 2005 that this drug was associated with a 30 percent increase in the risk of heart disease. Instead of acting immediately on this important information and warning patients of the potential risk, GSK took until June 2007, when a study was published in the *New England Journal of Medicine*, to bring this risk to light.[5] The lead researcher Steven Nissen, M.D., from the Cleveland Clinic, wrote in his report that both GlaxoSmithKline and the FDA should have taken (but didn't take) the necessary steps to adequately warn people using Avandia of the risks to their health. An examination of data from a pool of 42 studies provided by GSK showed that there was a 43 percent increase in the number of heart attacks and a 64 percent increase in the risk of dying from heart disease among people with type 2 diabetes taking Avandia, compared with people given a placebo. Keep in mind that the reason drugs are prescribed to lower blood sugar is to prevent the complications of diabetes, the most important of which is heart disease.

Given the facts that in 2006 alone, doctors in the United States wrote 13 million prescriptions for Avandia and that the results of this study were so damning, it is estimated that as many as 16,000 legal claims could be made against GSK in response to the study. But even though the FDA shares equal blame for allowing these deaths to happen, no legal action will be made against it.

▸ We have too many doctors. The ratio of practicing medical doctors to the population went from 151 doctors per 100,000 people in 1970 to 245 per 100,000 in 1992, an increase in ratio of 62 percent.

▸ We have too many medical specialists. Fifty years ago, specialists were 30 percent of the physician workforce; today, specialists account for 70 to 80 percent.

▶ There are too many unnecessary visits to doctors, medical procedures, surgeries, and drugs being administered by doctors. Currently, medical analysts estimate that 36 percent of physician visits are unnecessary, 56 percent of surgeries are unnecessary, 15 percent of hospital outpatient visits are unnecessary, and half of all time spent in hospitals is not medically indicated.

One of the most disturbing statistics is that there is a direct correlation between the ratio of surgeons in an area and the percentage of the local population receiving surgeries. One research study found that an area with 4.5 surgeons per 10,000 population experienced 940 operations per 10,000 whereas an area with 2.5 surgeons per 10,000 experienced 590 operations per 10,000.[6] In other words, when the concentration of surgeons doubles, so does the rate of surgeries. It makes sense, doesn't it? After all, these surgeons need to perform surgeries to cover overhead and maintain their desired income. The problem is apparently worse for especially expensive surgeries. For example, according to a noted Harvard cardiologist and published studies in the *Journal of the American Medical Association*, more than 80 percent of coronary angioplasty and bypass operations are not necessary.[7] These surgical procedures cost, on average, $40,000. The rise in expensive hospital-based procedures such as coronary artery bypass operations prescribed by highly specialized physicians is considered by health economists to be the primary cause of our escalating health care costs.

SELLING SICKNESS

As if it were not enough to gouge the pocketbooks of Americans for drugs to treat sickness, the drug companies have used their influence to narrow the boundaries of what is normal for conditions such as cholesterol and blood pressure, so that they can cast a bigger net and get doctors to prescribe their drugs to more patients. The goal of the drug companies is transparent and has been expertly revealed in *Selling Sickness: How the World's Biggest Pharmaceutical Companies Are Turning Us All into Patients*, by Ray Moynihan and Alan Cassells.

The ultimate strategy of Merck, one of the largest drug companies in the world, was outlined more than 30 years ago when Henry Gadsden, the head of Merck at the time, was interviewed by *Fortune* magazine. Gasden said he wanted Merck to be more like Wrigley gum, that it was his dream to make drugs for healthy people so that Merck could sell to everyone.[8] This dream is now nearly reality, if you take a look at the number of people currently taking statin medications to lower cholesterol. By the way, the first statin drug to be marketed was Merck's Mevocor (lovastatin).

Sales of statin drugs such as Lipitor, Crestor, and Pravachol have reached unbelievable heights; these are by far the best-selling category of drugs. How these drugs rose in popularity serves as a model for the entire drug industry and is explained in Chapter 7. One strategy of the drug com-

---

Selling Addiction

Oxycodone is a potent and highly addictive synthetic opiate-like pain medication marketed under the proprietary names Percocet, Combunox, Roxicodone, OxyContin, and as generic alternatives. Of these, the most notorious is OxyContin (the name is actually short for Oxycodone Continuous release) popularly referred to as "pharmaceutical heroin" and marketed as a miracle drug for people with chronic pain. On May 10, 2007, Purdue Pharma—the company that makes OxyContin—and three current and former executives pleaded guilty in a U.S. court to criminal charges that they misled regulators, doctors, and patients by falsely claiming that OxyContin was less addictive, less subject to abuse, and less likely to cause withdrawal symptoms than other pain medications. To resolve criminal and civil charges related to the drug's "misbranding," Purdue Frederick— the parent company of Purdue Pharma—and its top three executives agreed to pay about $634 million in fines and other charges, one of the largest amounts ever paid by a drug company in such a case. OxyContin was launched in 1995, and its annual sales reached approximately $2 billion prior to the arrival of generic products in 2004 and are still over $1 billion annually. So, although $634 million seems like a huge fine, it was still not as high as the drug company's profits.

panies selling statins was to expand the number of people who met the criterion of "high cholesterol." Every time the level of cholesterol considered "high" is lowered, millions of new customers are created overnight. Since the statins were introduced in 1987, the number of people in the United States with high cholesterol has increased from 13 million to nearly 100 million.

Who are these experts defining "high" cholesterol? Are they paid representatives of drug companies? It would seem so. Eight of the nine experts who wrote the latest cholesterol guidelines for the U.S. National Institutes of Health also serve as speakers, consultants, or researchers to the world's largest drug companies.[9] Most of the individual authors were receiving money from at least four companies, and one "expert" had taken money from ten.

DRUG COMPANIES CONTROL
MEDICAL EDUCATION

Believe it or not, most physicians receive very little formal education in nutrition, and also very little in pharmacology, the study of drug actions and effects. Doctors are taught general principles of pharmacology in medical school, but most of their understanding is derived from their hospital training with practicing physicians. How do those practicing physicians learn about pharmacology? From the drug companies, of course. The drug companies sponsor medical journals and educational programs, and there is roughly one drug company sales representative for every 10 doctors in America. Doctors rely on these sales reps for information about drugs, yet less than 5 percent of these sales reps have had formal training in pharmacology.

Detailed analysis has also shown that most physicians do not decide what drug to use on the basis of scientific research or cost; they base their decision almost entirely on the effectiveness of the drug company's marketing and advertising. In essence, doctors are often bribed or lied to so that they will prescribe certain medications. The bribing is well-known; the lying becomes apparent when we examine pharmaceutical advertisements and the manipulation of data in published studies. Here are some sobering facts:

- According to former editors of three major medical journals—the *Lancet*, the *New England Journal of Medicine*, and the *British Medical Journal*—some journals are just an extension of the marketing departments of major drug companies.[3, 10, 11]

- An entire issue of the *Journal of the American Medical Association* (JAMA) was dedicated to evaluating the quality of research. One telling statistic: it is estimated that 95 percent of medical studies in the most prestigious journals contain false or misleading statistics.[12]

- Many research studies in medical journals are sponsored by drug companies and ghostwritten. In one analysis, 40 of 44 articles (91 percent) were ghostwritten, and in 31 articles the ghostwriter, as identified, was a statistician (and you know what they say about statistics).[13]

DRUG COMPANIES FUND RESEARCH AS A MARKETING TOOL

The gold standard that physicians are taught to use in evaluating a drug's efficacy and safety is the randomized, controlled clinical trial designed to eliminate all aspects of chance to provide a statistical outcome. However, this gold standard has become fool's gold for several reasons. What the doctors usually don't know is that they are placing their faith in research whose outcomes are largely predetermined by the drug companies' careful stacking of the deck before the trial ever begins. The doctors do not realize that instead of using impartial, neutral research organizations, the drug companies hire for-profit contract research organizations to conduct their clinical trials.[14] And virtually all the clinical research done in the United States is designed to benefit the drug manufacturers, because they are paying for it. In

1980, research sponsored by drug companies accounted for about one-third of all clinical research done in the United States. By 2007 that proportion had grown to an estimated 90 percent.[15]

Drug companies are very smart—remember that they are the most profitable industry in the world—but the research organizations may even be smarter! They know that in order to be successful, they must be able to produce results that will make their customers very happy. So they must assure the clients that they will produce the best possible results; and if by chance a study does not produce the desired outcome, then that study will never be published. Even if a study is published, the research organizations often withhold important data. Perhaps one of the most celebrated examples of convenient omission is the case of Celebrex. The reason why Celebrex and Vioxx came into prominence was to avoid the ulcers caused by anti-inflammatory drugs such as aspirin and ibuprofen. The makers of Celebrex achieved this goal when the results of two six-month studies indicated that Celebrex caused fewer stomach problems than the older drugs. But what the drug company failed to disclose was that the two studies were actually for 12 and 15 months, respectively. The reason the results were published after only six months was that with longer use—12 months—there was actually no difference, with regard to ulcers, between Celebrex and the older drugs ibuprofen and Voltaren.[16, 17] In light of the subsequent disclosures about Celebrex and Vioxx, it would seem that should never have been approved for use (these drugs and their natural alternatives are discussed further in Chapter 5).

THE "OFF-LABEL" MARKET AND DRUG PROFITS

"Off-label use" of a drug refers to prescribing it for a purpose other than its FDA-approved use. In most cases, once the FDA allows a drug to be prescribed, doctors have the right to prescribe it as they deem fit. But although it is entirely legal in the United States for doctors to do this, it is illegal for drug companies to market off-label uses. Still, there are ways around this restriction. In fact, drug companies spend considerable resources to promote off-label uses.

The most notorious example of an off-label strategy involved the Parke-Davis division of Warner-Lambert (which was swallowed up by the drug giant Pfizer in 2000) and its drug Neurontin,[18] which had been approved for use in epilepsy that was unresponsive to other drugs alone. Parke-Davis constructed an elaborate illegal scheme to increase the profitability of Neurontin by promoting it for other uses. Publicly, Parke-Davis/Pfizer called the plan a "public relations strategy." Internal documents, however, detailed a well-orchestrated strategy to fund poorly designed studies for other uses such as anxiety, headaches, bipolar depression, and pain—conditions that affect much larger numbers of people than epilepsy does. Parke-Davis/Pfizer arranged for contract clinical research organizations to conduct the studies and then paid academic authors and experts to sign their names to the studies. Once published, these research articles were aggressively disseminated to physicians. Parke-Davis also sponsored educational meetings and conferences at which not only the presenters were paid: physicians in the audience were also paid to attend, or in some cases the meetings were, essentially, paid vacations for the doctors.

The strategy worked brilliantly, at least until 1996, when David Franklin, a Parke-Davis sales representative, blew the whistle on the operation. Even then, Neurontin's sales soared from $97.5 million in 1995 to nearly $2.7 billion in 2003. In 2004, Pfizer paid $430 million to the federal government to settle the case. This fine was hardly a deterrent; more than likely, it was built into the price of the drug.

WHY IS THERE A BIAS AMONG MEDICAL DOCTORS AGAINST ALTERNATIVE MEDICINE?

The simple answer to this important question is that many doctors are simply not educated in the value of nutrition and other natural therapies; in fact, most were told during their education to tell their patients that alternative medicines are worthless. Many doctors are not aware of, or choose to ignore the data on, beneficial natural therapies such as diet, exercise, and dietary supplements, even if the data are overwhelmingly positive. Rather than admit that they don't know, most doctors have a knee-jerk reaction: it can't be true. If they are not up on something, they will be down on it, to protect their own ego. They often suffer from what I call the "tomato effect." This is a reference to the belief, widely held in eighteenth-century North America, that tomatoes were poisonous, even though they were a dietary staple in Europe. It wasn't until 1820, when Robert Gibbon Johnson ate a tomato on the courthouse steps in Salem, Indiana, that the barrier against the "poisonous" tomato was broken in the minds of many Americans.

The attitude of many physicians toward alternative therapies is quite similar to the tomato effect. For example, diet is a fundamental aspect of health. But when patients ask about diet therapy or a nutritional supplement for a particular condition, even if the nutritional approach has considerable support in the scientific literature and this literature proves its safety and effectiveness, most doctors will caution their patients against taking the natural route or will tell them that it will not help, though it won't hurt either. The truth is that in many cases, the doctor just doesn't know anything about it. There is more to this story; I will discuss it in Chapter 10 and will also point out that:

- ▸ It took the medical community more than 40 years to accept the link between low levels of folic acid in pregnant women and neural-tube defects in newborns. It is estimated that 70 to 85 percent of more than 100,000 cases of spina bifida in children born during that time could have been prevented if doctors had not been so biased against scientific data on nutritional supplements.[19]

- ▸ The true number of adverse drug reactions (ADRs) may be even more than 2 million per year, because ADRs are underreported to the FDA (reporting is a voluntary program). For example, the FDA receives an average of 80 reports each year about adverse reactions caused by the drug digoxin; however, a systematic survey of Medicare records indicates that approximately 30,000 hospital admissions each year are for digoxin toxicity.[20]

- ▸ In the worst-case scenario, over the last 20 years ephedra and other natural products were linked to approximately 150 deaths (virtually all of which were related to excessive dosage or abuse). In contrast, over the last 20 years approximately 2 million people in the United States died from adverse drug reactions; these deaths included more than 300,000 caused by aspirin and other NSAIDs.[21]

HEALTH CARE VERSUS DISEASE MANAGEMENT

Talk of health care reform is everywhere. It's was the hot political topic of the 1990s. For good reason, the cost of health care in America is wildly out of control. However, fundamentally, what is being debated is not "health care" reform but the reform of "disease management." The U.S. system is not devoted to promoting health. It is obsessed with managing disease. In fact, the combined influence of the pharmaceutical industry, the FDA, and public policy has taken "health care" virtually out of our system.

Everything in our system depends on people's getting sick. The basic treatments covered by medical insurance revolve around patented pharmaceutical drugs, designed to suppress the symptoms of disease, and expensive surgeries. No one involved in the medical industry really wants to see true health care reform. Managing disease is simply too big and too lucrative a business. This might make sense if Americans were getting their money's worth. But although drug companies, doctors, insurance companies, and hospitals are pulling in big money, the medical approach promoted by these interests is not necessarily helping people get well. True health and healing require personal responsibility, fundamental support, and removal of obstacles to health.

If the focus in medicine were on promoting health and wellness—if this became the dominant medical model—not only would health care costs be drastically reduced, but the health of Americans would improve dramatically. It is a sad fact that while we are grossly outspending every other nation in the world on health care, we are not, as a nation, healthy individuals. National health surveys have shown that almost half of all working Americans either have a serious chronic disease (arthritis, heart disease, high blood pressure, cancer, gallbladder disease, diabetes, rheumatism, emphysema, serious arteriosclerosis, and so on) or are in poor health. The health of their nonworking dependents is even worse: half to two-thirds of these adults suffer from chronic disease (such as cancer, diabetes, and heart disease) and generally poor health. What's especially alarming about these statistics is that these are adults supposedly in their prime. The situation is worse for the elderly, virtually all of whom suffer from one or more chronic degenerative diseases.

Percentage of Adult Americans Suffering from the 10 Most Common Chronic Diseases [22]

Condition	MEN, BY AGE			WOMEN, BY AGE		
	18–44	45–64	65+	18–44	45–64	65+
Arthritis	4.1%	21.4%	38.3%	6.4%	33.9%	54.4%
Asthma, emphysema, and chronic bronchitis	5.5	8.8	16.7	9.3	11.4	12.6
Cancer	0.2	2.3	5.2	0.5	2.2	3.8
Chronic sinusitis	13.6	16.3	14.1	18.3	19.9	17.0
Diabetes	0.8	5.1	9.1	1.0	5.7	9.9
Hay fever	10.3	7.9	NA*	12.1	9.8	NA*
Hearing impairment	6.3	19.6	36.2	4.0	10.6	26.8
High blood pressure	6.6	25.4	32.7	5.7	27.4	45.6
Ischemic heart disease	0.3	8.7	17.9	0.3	4.3	12.1
Visual impairment	4.3	6.2	10.4	1.7	3.2	18.8

* NA = data not available.

WELLNESS-ORIENTED MEDICINE IS THE SOLUTION

Wellness-oriented medicine, such as naturopathic medicine, provides a realistic solution to escalating health care costs and poor health status in the United States. Equally important, this orientation can increase patients' satisfaction. Studies have observed that patients who take the natural medicine–health promotion approach are more satisfied with the results of their treatment than they were with the results of conventional treatments such as drugs and surgeries. A few studies have directly compared patients' satisfaction with natural medicine and patients' satisfaction with conventional medicine. The largest study was done in the Netherlands, where natural medicine practitioners are an integral part of the health care system. This extensive study compared satisfaction in 3,782 patients who were seeing either a conventional physician or a "complementary practitioner." The patients seeing the practitioner of natural medicine reported better results for almost every condition. Of particular interest was the observation that the patients seeing the complementary practitioners were somewhat sicker at the start of therapy, and that in only four of the 23 conditions did the conventional medical patients report better results.

Patient Satisfaction with Complementary Practitioners Compared with Medical Specialists

Symptom	Complementary Practitioner, Patients Improved, Percent	Medical Specialist, Patients Improved, Percent
Palpitations	63	59
Stiffness	67	54
Feeling very ill	75	78
Itching or burning	71	50
Tiredness or lethargy	70	60
Fever	86	100
Pain	70	58
Tension or depression	69	65
Coughing	76	50
Blood loss	100	100
Tingling, numbness	59	40
Shortness of breath	77	53
Nausea and vomiting	71	67
Diarrhea and constipation	67	50
Poor vision or hearing	31	47
Paralysis	80	67

(*continued on next page*)

Symptom	Complementary Practitioner, Patients Improved, Percent	Medical Specialist, Patients Improved, Percent
Insomnia	58	45
Dizziness and fainting	80	53
Anxiety	65	64
Skin rash	58	50
Emotional instability	56	63
Sexual problems	57	57
Other	75	56

FINAL COMMENTS

In communicating with patients and my audiences I have learned that people process new information by asking themselves the question "What does this info have to do with me?" What I have done in this chapter is raise the issue of trust. In the forthcoming chapters, I will give more specific examples of why we should not be led blindly into using drugs or undergoing surgery without first asking some important questions:

What is the real benefit of taking this drug?

What are the risks of either taking or not taking the drug?

Are there any effective alternatives?

I also want to point out that although we all have some common characteristics, we also have our own unique biochemistry. Unfortunately, what might be a great medicine for one person might not work for or may even cause harm in someone else. Biochemical individuality is discussed in more depth in Chapter 11.

2

THE NUMBER ONE THING
THAT THEY DON'T WANT
YOU TO KNOW

*"Nature is doing her best each moment to make us well.
She exists for no other end. Do not resist. With the
least inclination to be well, we should not be sick."*
—Henry David Thoreau

THE MOST IMPORTANT SECRET that the drug companies don't want known is something that most physicians have long forgotten: we all have an absolutely astounding capacity to heal ourselves. Perhaps, of all nature's miracles, the human mind and body are the most amazing. As Thoreau realized, nature works constantly to ensure that your body functions well. Health is our natural state.

One fundamental principle of naturopathic medicine is the body's innate ability to spontaneously heal itself. Recently, as an exercise, I took a look at popular conventional medical textbooks for evidence of this idea of self-healing. Surprisingly, the word "healing" was not found in any of the indexes, and except for the description of a disease as being "self-limited," I found no evidence of self-healing other than an occasional mention of the "placebo response." Undoubtedly you have heard of this term. A placebo contains no medicinal agent, yet these "sugar pills" and other sham treatments often produce tremendous effects.

Now, I am not saying that any condition should be treated with a placebo. I am only giving examples in this chapter to illustrate a point: conventional medicine fails to recognize the tremendous healing power within us. That said, I do want to make another critical point: many drugs and conventional treatments elicit little more than a placebo response, while at the same time potentially producing unwanted side effects.

THE CURIOUS CASE OF KREBIOZEN

One of the more dramatic examples of the placebo effect reported in medical literature involved a patient of Dr. Bruno Klopfer, a researcher who participated in testing the drug Krebiozen in 1950.[1] Krebiozen had received sensational national publicity as a "cure" for cancer. These reports caught the eye of a man with advanced cancer—a lymphosarcoma. The patient, Mr. Wright, had huge tumor masses throughout his body and was in such desperate physical condition that he frequently had to take oxygen by mask and fluid had to be removed from his chest every two days. When the patient learned that Dr. Klopfer was involved in research on Krebiozen, he begged to be treated with it. Dr. Klopfer agreed, and the patient's recovery was startling—"The tumor masses had melted like snowballs on a hot stove, and in only a few days, they were half their original size!" The injections were continued until Mr. Wright was discharged from the hospital and had resumed a full, normal life, a complete reversal of his disease and its grim prognosis.

However, within two months of his recovery, a report that Krebiozen was not effective was leaked to the press. Learning of this report, Mr. Wright quickly began to revert to his former condition. Suspicious about the patient's relapse, his doctors decided to take advantage of the opportunity to test the dramatic regenerative capabilities of the mind. The patient was told that a new version of Krebiozen had been developed, that it overcame the difficulties described in the press, and that he would be given some of it as soon as it could be procured.

With much pomp and ceremony, which increased the patient's expectations to a fever pitch, a saline water placebo was injected. Recovery from this second nearly terminal state was even more dramatic than that from the first. Mr. Wright's tumor masses melted, his chest fluid vanished, and he became a picture of health. The saline water injections were continued, since they had worked wonders. He then remained symptom-free for over two months. At this time the final AMA announcement appeared in the press—"nationwide tests show Krebiozen to be a worthless drug in the treatment of cancer." Within a few days of this report, Mr. Wright was re-admitted to the hospital in dire straits. His faith now gone, his last hope vanished, he died two days later.

WHAT IS THE PLACEBO RESPONSE?

Is a placebo response all in a person's mind? Absolutely not! What recent re-search demonstrates is that the placebo response is a complex phenome-non, initiated by the mind and leading to a cascade of real, measurable effects. In few words, the placebo response is the activation of the healing centers of our being in a way that produces profound physiological changes. The body has two internal mechanisms to maintain health. The first is the inherent internal healing mechanism: the vital force, chi; or the primitive life support and repair mechanism that operates even in a person who is asleep, unconscious, or comatose. The second mechanism involves the power of the mind and emotions to intervene and affect the course of health and disease in a way that enhances or supersedes the body's innate vital force. The placebo response seems to involve activation of the higher control center, but this does not mean that its effects are solely in the mind.

One of the leading researchers into the placebo response is Dr. Fabrizio Benedetti of the University of Turin in Italy. He has conducted some very detailed studies trying to discover its underlying features.[2] For example, nu-merous studies have documented that the pain-relieving effects of a placebo are mediated by endorphins—the body's own morphine-like substances. Clinical studies have shown that in roughly 56 percent of patients a placebo saline injection is as effective as morphine against severe pain, and this pain relief can be completely nullified by adding naloxone, a drug that blocks the effects of morphine, to the saline injection. As a result of such experiments, a great deal of the credit for the placebo response has been given to endorphins, but Dr. Benedetti's research has shown that a placebo can produce much more profound changes than increasing endorphin levels. For example, he has shown that a saline placebo can reduce tremors and muscle stiffness in people with Parkinson's disease. That is not surprising, perhaps; but he also found, very interestingly that when the placebo produced noticeable improvements in symptoms, there was a simultaneous significant change in the measured activity of neurons in the patients' brains, as shown by a brain scan. In particular, as the researchers administered the saline, they found that individual neurons in the subthalamic nucleus (a common target for surgical attempts to relieve the symptoms of Parkinson's disease) began to fire less often and with fewer "bursts"—a characteristic feature associated with Parkinsonian tremors. Somehow the saline placebo resulted in the processing of the information by healing centers in the brain to specifically target an effect that would reduce the dysfunction in the areas of the brain affected by Parkinson's disease.

Other studies have shown demonstrable changes in brain activity through modern imaging techniques (e.g., CAT scans and MRIs) in other disease states with the placebo response as well as the experience of different emotions. For example, one study showed that expectation or hope is able to stimulate the part of the brain that is activated by pain medications and is associated with relief of pain. In addition, numerous changes in chemical mediators of pain, inflammation, and mood have also been demonstrated with the placebo response. There is tremendous evidence, then, that the placebo response is a highly specific and precisely targeted healing effect, triggered by conscious and unconscious centers in the brain. Rather than discounting and trying to avoid a placebo response, modern medicine should be more intent on developing techniques and practices designed to stimulate the healing centers within patients that have been noted in these studies with placebos.[3]

THE PLACEBO RESPONSE IN
MEDICAL RESEARCH

The development of the drug industry has been based largely on the perceived value of the placebo-controlled trial. In order for a drug to be approved, it must show a therapeutic effect greater than that of a placebo. Because both the doctor's and the patient's belief in the value of a treatment can affect the outcome, most placebo-controlled trials are usually double-blind: that is, not only the patients but also the doctors are unaware of who is receiving a placebo. Nearly all double-blind studies show some benefit in the placebo group. For example, in 1955 the researcher H. K. Beecher published a groundbreaking paper, "The Powerful Placebo," in which he concluded that, across the 26 studies he analyzed, an average of 32 percent of patients responded to a placebo.[4] It is generally thought that the overall placebo response is about 32 percent in clinical trials (this average is based on Beecher's work and studies), but there is evidence that for some conditions it may be as high as 80 to 90 percent in actual clinical practice. The reason is that in the real world, the placebo response is enhanced by both the doctor's and the patient's expectations.

Conditions That Have Been Associated with a High Response to a Placebo

Angina	Depression
Anxiety	Diabetes (type 2)
Arthritis	Drug dependence
Asthma	Dyspepsia
Behavioral problems	Gastric ulcers
Claudication, intermittent	Hay fever
Common cold	Headaches
Cough, chronic	Hypertension

Insomnia   Nausea of pregnancy

Labor and postpartum pain   Pain

Menstrual cramps   Psychoneuroses

Premenstrual syndrome   Tremor

Ménière's disease

BASIC COMPONENTS OF THE
PLACEBO RESPONSE

The noted Harvard psychologist Herbert Benson has described three basic components of heightening a placebo response: one, the belief and expectation of the patient; two, the belief and expectation of the physician; three, the interaction between the physician and the patient. When these three are in concert, the placebo effect is greatly magnified. Benson believes that the placebo effect yields beneficial clinical results in 60 to 90 percent of diseases.[5] He states that the placebo "has been one of medicine's most potent assets and it should not be belittled or ridiculed. Unlike most other treatments, it is safe and inexpensive and has withstood the test of time." I agree with him completely.

As powerful as the placebo response is, it still requires activation. If the therapeutic interaction between the physician and the patient does not stimulate the patient's hope, faith, and belief, the chances of success are measurably diminished no matter how strong or effective the medication may be. It has been repeatedly demonstrated in clinical trials designed to better understand the placebo effect that the beliefs of both the patient and the doctor, and their trust in each other and the process, generate a significant portion of the therapeutic results.

Conventional medicine often criticizes and belittles therapies that have not been stringently tested using the double-blind, placebo-controlled trial, but it is arguing against something that has been time-tested—the art of healing. A compassionate, warm, caring physician will produce better outcomes and encounter fewer side effects with medications than a cold, uncaring, uninterested, emotionless physician.

THE OPPOSITE OF A PLACEBO

The term "placebo" comes from the Latin for "I will please." Its opposite is a nocebo, from the Latin for "I will harm." The nocebo effect is a side effect from an apparently inert substance or a sham treatment. Healthy individuals have adverse effects from a placebo about 25 percent of the time, and if patients are specifically asked about adverse effects, the proportion can rise to 70 percent. "Nocebo response" usually describes an adverse reaction to a placebo, but the term could also be applied to an unusual or exaggerated adverse response to a medication. Does that mean that a nocebo effect is not real? Not at all; it is just as real as the real thing.[6]

Symptoms and Side Effects Produced by Placebos

Anger	Headache
Anorexia	Lightheadedness
Behavioral changes	Pain
Depression	Palpitation
Dermatitis	Pupillary dilation
Diarrhea	Rash
Drowsiness	Weakness
Hallucinations	

THE POWER OF EXPECTATIONS

Just as the placebo response is influenced by a patient's attitude, so too is the nocebo response. It is another example of the power of expectations.

The classic example comes from the Framingham Heart Study, in which, among women with similar risk factors, those who believed they were prone to heart disease were four times more likely to die from a heart attack.[7] Expectations are influenced by many factors (including price), all of which play a role in establishing the patient's level of faith.

Definitions of Some Expectation Effects Behind the Placebo Response

Hawthorne effect	Subjects respond to knowledge of being evaluated and observed.
Jastrow effect	Subjects respond to explicit expectation about outcome.
Pygmalion effect	Evaluators expect therapeutic benefit, so they see it.
John Henry effect	Control subjects attempt to emulate expected outcomes.
Halo effect	Subjects respond to novelty of treatment (i.e., new technology).
Experiment effect	Evaluators consciously (or not) interpret outcomes differently.
Socialization effect	Others reporting benefit influence outcomes.
Value effect	Price of treatment influences expected outcomes.

THE ROLE OF FAITH AND SPIRITUALITY IN MEDICINE

It is amazing to me that most physicians ignore one of the most powerful healing techniques known. Prayer costs nothing, has no negative side effects, and fits perfectly into any treatment plan. No matter what faith you embrace, you can use the power of prayer to lead you to better health—of body, mind, and soul.

Most physicians are taught that any consideration of religious commitment is beyond the legitimate interest and scope of medical care. It should not be this way, but many of them believe that faith and medical science are mutually exclusive, despite the fact that numerous scientific studies have now fully validated the efficacy of faith, prayer, and religion in healing.[8, 9]

In addition, patients know that prayer works. In 1996 *USA Today* conducted a poll of 1,000 American adults; 79 percent of the respondents endorsed the belief that spiritual faith and prayer can help people recover from disease, and 63 percent agreed that physicians should talk to patients about spiritual faith and prayer.[10] Indeed, my feeling is that it is medically irresponsible *not* to include a spiritual dimension in a patient's plan for treatment and recovery.

One of the leaders who brought the healing power of prayer to the forefront was Larry Dossey, M.D., author of the best-selling books *Healing Words: The Power of Prayer and the Practice of Medicine* (HarperCollins, 1993) and *Prayer Is Good Medicine* (HarperCollins, 1996). In these books, Dr. Dossey provides a thorough review of the scientific evidence. Not surprisingly, he found that prayer has received relatively little attention from the research community. His systematic analysis of more than 4.3 million published reports indexed on Medline (the U.S. Government's medical database) from 1980 to 1996 found only 364 studies that included faith, religion, or prayer as part of the treatment. The numbers are small, but the conclusion is huge: the data show that prayer and religious commitment promote good health and healing.

Scientific investigation into the healing power of prayer has shown than it can affect physical processes in a variety of organisms. Specifically, studies have explored the effects of prayer on humans and on nonhuman subjects, including water, enzymes, bacteria, fungi, yeast, red blood cells, cancer cells, pacemaker cells, seeds, plants, algae, moth larvae, mice, and chicks. In these studies, prayer affected how these organisms grew or functioned. What scientists discovered—no doubt to their amazement—is that prayer affected a number of biological processes, including:

- Enzyme activity
- Growth rates of leukemic white blood cells
- Mutation rates of bacteria
- Germination and growth rates of various seeds
- Firing rate of pacemaker cells
- Healing rates of wounds
- Size of goiters and tumors
- Time required to awaken from anesthesia
- Autonomic effects such as electrodermal activity of the skin
- Hemoglobin levels

In my opinion, given the scientific support for the beneficial effects of prayer, *not* praying for the best possible outcome may be the equivalent of deliberately withholding an effective drug or surgical procedure.

If praying is good for others, can we do it for ourselves? Absolutely. Dr. Benson of Harvard found that patients who prayed or meditated evoked their body's relaxation response.[11] This response—the exact opposite of the stress response, the "fight or flight" reaction that we feel during tense situations—includes decreases in heart rate, breathing rate, muscle tension, and sometimes even blood pressure. The medical implications of the relaxation response are enormous and may serve as the basis for most mind-body techniques such as guided imagery (discussed below) and meditation. The relaxation response has been shown to produce useful effects in a variety of different disease states. For example, cancer patients who undergo chemotherapy treatment and who learn to evoke the relaxation response are significantly less likely to experience nausea and fatigue.

Creating the Relaxation Response

Here is a simple exercise we use with many of our cancer patients to help them achieve the relaxation response, and program white blood cells to destroy tumors. The exercise will improve your ability to breathe from the diaphragm, achieve the relaxation response, and reduce stress. Practice the following for at least five minutes, twice a day.

▸ Find a quiet, comfortable place to sit or lie down.

▸ Place your feet slightly apart and find a comfortable position for your arms.

▸ Inhale through your nose and exhale through your mouth.

▸ Concentrate on your breathing.

▸ Inhale while slowly counting to four. Notice with each breath you take that you are breathing effortlessly by using your diaphragm. You should feel as if the air is expanding first into your abdomen and then up into your lungs, and then that warmth is expanding to all parts of your body.

▸ Pause for one second, then slowly exhale to a count of four. As you exhale, your abdomen should move inward. As the air flows out, feel of the tension and stress leaving your body.

▸ As you begin to relax, clear your mind of any distractions by imagining a peaceful, healing environment. Bathe yourself in the feeling of love.

▸ Begin to focus on the location of the cancer. Imagine that your white blood cells are flowing into the area and, like the little Pac-Men they are, eating the cancer away.

▸ Repeat the process for five to ten minutes or until you achieve a sense of deep relaxation.

If you find yourself having trouble learning how to relax or perform visualization exercises, we recommend contacting the Academy for Guided Imagery (1-800-726-2070) or visiting its Web site (http://www.interactive imagery.com) to find a practitioner who specializes in guided imagery. You can also ask your doctor for a referral. Taking a yoga class is also a great way to learn how to breathe with your diaphragm and learn how to relax.

RELIGION AND THE HEART

Researcher Jeff Levin, Ph.D., author of *God, Faith, and Health*, is recognized as one of the leading researchers in spirituality and health. As a first-year graduate student in the School of Public Health at the University of North Carolina in Chapel Hill, Levin became intrigued by two articles that found a surprising and significant connection between spirituality and heart disease, a connection that remains one of the best-researched areas of the positive effects of religious behavior on health. His curiosity led to an in-depth evaluation and pioneering research on the impact of religious practices on disease.[12] In *God, Faith, and Health*, Dr. Levin notes that there are more than 50 studies in which religious practices were found to be protective against cardiovascular disease, including death due to heart attacks and strokes as well as against numerous risk factors such as high blood pressure and elevated cholesterol and triglyceride levels. In particular, Dr. Levin highlights the strong inverse correlation between strong religious commitment and blood pressure that was evident no matter what religion an individual chose to practice or his or her geographical location or ancestry.

FINAL COMMENTS

Often, I am asked for a blueprint for good health and effective healing. Most people are looking for a simple answer, but my feeling is that living healthfully requires a truly comprehensive commitment in all aspects of being. Here are what I consider the critical steps to vibrant health:

▸ Step 1—Incorporate spirituality in your life.

▸ Step 2—Develop a positive mental attitude.

▸ Step 3—Focus on establishing positive relationships.

▸ Step 4—Follow a healthy lifestyle.

- Step 5—Be active and get regular physical exercise.

- Step 6—Eat a health-promoting diet.

- Step 7—Support your body through proper nutritional supplementation and body work.

  These steps are explained fully in Chapter 11.

3

AN OVERLOOKED GOAL
OF HEALING—REMOVING
OBSTACLES TO A CURE

*"The art of healing comes from nature, not from
the physician. Therefore the physician must
start from nature, with an open mind."*
—Paracelsus

ONE FUNDAMENTAL PRINCIPLE OF naturopathic medicine, as well as of other time-tested systems of medicine, is to first remove obstacles to a cure. It makes sense, but it is a principle that is seldom followed in conventional modern medicine. What do I mean by obstacles to a cure? Well, a nutrient deficiency is often a serious obstacle to true healing. In addition, there are factors such as habitual expression of anger, contamination with heavy metals or environmental toxins, genetic predispositions, metabolic abnormalities, and obesity. These obstacles often make even the most powerful medicines—whether natural or man-made—ineffective.

To illustrate the importance of removing obstacles to healing, let me tell you about my patient, Carl, who was 52 years old and worked in the men's clothing department at Nordstroms. He came to see me for help in getting his high blood pressure under control. He told me he was frustrated with the "medical world" and absolutely hated the drugs his doctors had prescribed. The side effects (dizziness, tingling sensations, and numbness in his hands and feet—not to mention impotence) were driving him nuts. Worse, the treatment did not seem to be getting his blood pressure down. His typical reading was 150/105 (a normal reading is closer to 120/80).

Carl did not fit the mold of the usual patient with high blood pressure. First of all, he was not overweight: in fact, he was in great shape. He was an avid runner and ate a health-promoting diet. Except for his high blood pressure and some frequent headaches, he considered himself to be in excellent physical health.

The medical literature and my clinical experience taught me that a patient like Carl, who doesn't fit the typical profile, may have high levels of body lead. Several studies have found that lead raises blood pressure by negatively affecting kidney function.

Because I know that people who live in large cities or areas with "soft" water typically have higher lead levels, I asked Carl where he lived. He replied that he had "a nice old house right above a major freeway in downtown Seattle." He also told me that he ran 20-plus miles a week, mostly on a busy road along the Seattle waterfront. His route was picturesque, but I was sure that he was sucking in too much pollution. I had the nurse collect a sample of Carl's hair so that we could send it out for a hair mineral analysis (hair analysis is a very good screening test for heavy-metal toxicity).

I was shocked by the results. Carl's lead levels were literally off the chart. Despite these high levels, Carl was unaffected by symptoms commonly seen in people with high chronic lead exposure, including depression and neurological complaints such as visual disturbances.

For some patients with high lead levels I will recommend intravenous chelation therapy. This process involves slowly infusing ethylenediaminetetraacetic acid (EDTA), an amino-acid-like molecule, into the bloodstream. There, EDTA chelates (binds with) minerals such as calcium, iron, copper, and lead and carries them to the kidneys to be excreted. Intravenous (IV) EDTA chelation has been commonly used for lead poisoning, and it is also used for treating patients with atherosclerosis (hardening of the arteries).

In Carl's case, though, I thought oral (as opposed to IV) chelation might work to reduce his lead levels. I was optimistic because although Carl consumed a healthy diet, he did not take any nutritional supplements. I felt that we could "get the lead out" and lower his blood pressure simply by flooding his body with the nutrients it was starving for: calcium, magnesium, and zinc, as well as vitamins such as C, E, and the B vitamins. I also prescribed a garlic extract equal to four cloves of fresh garlic daily, but without the odor.

I thought that, for the time being, Carl should continue to take his prescribed blood pressure medication: Atenolol (a beta-blocker) and hydrochlorothiazide (a diuretic). But I urged him to monitor his blood pressure carefully. The extra calcium and magnesium he would be putting into his system can in some cases cause blood pressure to drop too low when a patient is on these medications.

Carl's blood pressure slowly started coming down after about a month. By the end of two months he needed only half the dosage of Atenolol, and after three months he was totally off the drug. At his last visit with me, Carl's blood pressure had dropped to 110/70. He still runs, but I persuaded him to change his route. The view is still spectacular—but instead of lead, he's inhaling a fresh sea breeze.

THE ROLE OF HEAVY METALS AS AN OBSTACLE TO A CURE

The toxic metals aluminum, arsenic, cadmium, lead, mercury, and nickel are often referred to as heavy metals, to distinguish them from the nutritional minerals, such as calcium and magnesium. Heavy metals tend to accumulate within the brain, kidneys, immune system, and other body tissues, where they can severely disrupt normal function.

The typical person living in the United States has more heavy metals in the body than is compatible with good health. For example, it is conservatively estimated that up to 25 percent of the U.S. population suffers from heavy metal poisoning to some extent.

Most of the heavy metals in the body are a result of environmental contamination due to industry. In the United States alone, industrial sources and leaded gasoline each year dump more than 600,000 tons of lead into the atmosphere to be inhaled or—after being deposited on food crops, in fresh water, and in soil—to be ingested. Other common sources of heavy metals include lead from the solder in tin cans, pesticide sprays, and cooking utensils; cadmium and lead from cigarette smoke; mercury from dental fillings, contaminated fish, and cosmetics; and aluminum from antacids and cookware. Professions with extremely high exposure include battery makers, gasoline station attendants, printers, roofers, solderers, dentists, and jewelers.

Sources of Heavy Metals and Symptoms Associated with Toxicity

Heavy Metal	Primary Sources	Linked to
Aluminum	Aluminum-containing antacids; aluminum cookware; drinking water	Alzheimer's disease; dementia; behavioral disorders; impaired brain function
Arsenic	Drinking water	Fatigue; headaches; heart disease and strokes; nerve disorders; anemia; Raynaud's phenomenon
Cadmium	Cigarette smoke; drinking water	Fatigue; impaired concentration and memory; high blood pressure; loss of smell; anemia; dry skin; prostate cancer; kidney problems
Lead	Cigarette smoke; car exhaust; dolomite, bone meal, and oyster shell calcium supplements; drinking water	Fatigue; headache; insomnia; nerve disorders; high blood pressure; attention deficit disorder; learning disabilities; anemia
Mercury	Amalgams (silver fillings); drinking water; fish and shellfish;	Fatigue; headache; insomnia; nerve disorders; high blood pressure; impaired memory and concentration
Nickel	Air and water	Heart disease; immune system dysfunction; allergies

Early signs of heavy metal poisoning are usually vague and depend on the level of toxicity. Mild cases of toxicity may be associated with headache, fatigue, and impaired ability to think or concentrate. As toxicity increases, so does the severity of signs and symptoms. A person with severe toxicity may also experience muscle pains, indigestion, tremors, constipation, anemia, pallor, dizziness, and poor coordination.

Numerous studies have demonstrated a strong relationship between intelligence, childhood learning disabilities, and body stores of lead, aluminum, cadmium, and mercury.[1, 2, 3, 4] Basically, the higher children's level of heavy metals, the lower their IQ. The same sort of relationship exists with blood pressure, as high blood pressure is also associated with higher levels of lead and other heavy metals.[5, 6] Heavy metals have a very strong affinity for body tissues composed of fat, like the brain, nerves, and kidneys. As a result, heavy metals are almost always linked to disturbances in mood and brain function as well as neurological problems (including multiple sclerosis) and high blood pressure (the kidneys regulate blood pressure).

DETERMINATION OF HEAVY-METAL TOXICITY

Hair mineral analysis is a valuable assessment tool that measures the levels of essential minerals as well as toxic heavy metals using a small sample of hair.[7] Hair mineral analysis is valuable for two reasons: (1) minerals play an extremely important role in human health, and (2) heavy metals such as lead, mercury, and aluminum can play an underlying role in many diseases, especially high blood pressure and neurological disease.

Hair levels of minerals and toxins correlate well with levels found in our organs as a result of exposure in the bloodstream. In a process called keratinization, hair develops just below the surface of the scalp and hardens once it breaks through. The minerals and heavy metals that run through your system accumulate in your hair over periods of time and become enclosed in the hair, allowing for a good reading of the levels of minerals and toxins in your body.

Anyone who is interested in optimal health can benefit from hair mineral assessment. This recommendation is particularly true if you have been exposed to any of the heavy metals or have symptoms associated with heavy metal toxicity.

Hair mineral analysis kits are available through many nutritionally oriented physicians as well as directly to consumers in many health food stores and online at www.bodybalance.com. The hair mineral analysis kits from BodyBalance that I recommend contain easy-to-follow instructions on how to collect the small sample of hair needed, a prepaid mailer to send the sample in, and a detailed interpretation and educational guide.

THE IMPORTANCE OF DETOXIFICATION

Heavy metals are just one type of chemical toxin that can cause an obstacle to healing. There are many others. Toxins can damage the body in insidious and cumulative ways. Once the detoxification system becomes overloaded, toxic metabolites accumulate, and can wreak havoc on our normal metabolic processes.

Besides heavy metals the long list of potential toxic chemicals includes drugs, alcohol, solvents, formaldehyde, pesticides, herbicides, and food additives. These toxic chemicals can give rise to a number of symptoms and are associated with an increased risk of certain cancers. They are particularly harmful to the brain and nervous system and can produce such symptoms as depression, headaches, mental confusion, mental illness, tingling in the hands and feet, abnormal nerve reflexes, and other signs of impaired nervous system function.

Toxins produced by bacteria and yeast in the gut can also significantly disrupt body functions and have been implicated in a wide variety of diseases including liver diseases, Crohn's disease, ulcerative colitis, thyroid disease, psoriasis, lupus, pancreatitis, allergies, asthma, and immune disorders.

Just a Few of the Thousands of Chemicals
Detectable in Every Living Human

- ▸ Toxic metals (lead, cadmium, mercury, arsenic, others)

- ▸ Polycyclic aromatic hydrocarbons (charbroiled meats)

- ▸ Volatile organic compounds (solvents)

- ▸ Tobacco smoke by-products (more than 500 potential chemicals)

- ▸ Phthalates (plastics)

- Acrylamides (french fries, bread)

- Dioxins, furans, PBDEs (fire retardants), and polychlorinated biphenyls (PCBs)

- Organochlorine by-products of water "purification"

- Organophosphate pesticides

- Organochlorine pesticides

- Carbamate pesticides

- Herbicides

- Pest repellents and disinfectants

DO YOU NEED TO DETOXIFY?

Have you ever noticed that many people treat their cars better than their bodies? They wouldn't dream of ignoring a warning light on the dashboard for an oil change or regular maintenance, but they often ignore the telltale signs that their body is in dire need of critical support. What are some of the body's warning signs? If you answer yes to any of the following questions, you definitely need to tune up your detoxification processes.

- Do you feel that you are not as healthy and vibrant as other people your age?

- Do you have low energy?

- Do you often have difficulty thinking clearly?

- Do you often feel blue or depressed?

- Do you get more than one or two colds a year?

- Do you suffer from premenstrual syndrome, fibrocystic breast disease, or uterine fibroids?

- Do you have sore achy muscles for no particular reason?

Is improving detoxification really an effective way to deal with these symptoms? In most cases, the answer is absolutely yes, as these symptoms often reflect nothing more than a squeaky wheel in need of maintenance. Also, as toxic metabolites accumulate, we become progressively more sensitive to other chemicals, some of which are not normally toxic.

If we reduce the toxic load on the body and give the body proper nutritional support, in most cases these bothersome symptoms will disappear. Even more important, by addressing these warning signs now we can ensure better long-term health and avoid the progression of minor problems to more serious conditions.

GUIDE TO INTERNAL CLEANSING

The concepts of internal cleansing and detoxification have been around for quite some time, but their critical role in promoting health has never been more important than it is now. We are exposed to an ever-increasing amount of toxic compounds in air, water, and food. I am amazed that there is literally no focus in conventional medicine on an individual's ability to detoxify substances as a factor determining overall health.

The body eliminates toxins either by directly neutralizing them or by excreting them in the urine or feces (and to a lesser degree from the lungs and skin). Toxins that the body is unable to eliminate build up in the tissues, typically in our fat stores. The liver, intestines, and kidneys are the primary organs of detoxification.

A rational approach to aiding the body's detoxification involves: (1) eating a diet that emphasizes fresh fruits and vegetables, whole grains, legumes, nuts, and seeds; (2) adopting a healthy lifestyle, including exercising regularly and avoiding alcohol; (3) taking a high-potency multiple vitamin and mineral supplement; (4) ingesting enough water to produce urination at least once every two and a half to three waking hours; and (5) going on a focused internal cleansing program at least once a year.

Fasting is often used as a detoxification method. Fasting is defined as abstinence from all food and drink except water or juice for a specific period of time, usually for a therapeutic or religious purpose. Although therapeutic fasting is probably one of the oldest known therapies, it has been largely ignored by the medical community, despite the fact that there is significant scientific research on fasting in the medical literature. Numerous medical journals have published articles on fasting in the treatment of obesity, chemical poisoning, rheumatoid arthritis, allergies, psoriasis, eczema, thrombophlebitis, leg ulcers, irritable bowel syndrome, impaired or deranged appetite, bronchial asthma, depression, neurosis, and schizophrenia.

However, in this day and age I do not recommend traditional fasting. The reason is that the toxins we are most concerned about are fat-soluble. When people fast or severely restrict their calorie intake, fat cells start to break down and release all the stored toxins. As a result, there can be a tremendous increase in circulating toxins, and without the right support these toxic substances can be redistributed into our organs, especially our brain and kidneys.

So, what I recommend instead is a focused internal cleansing program like the Seven-Day Total Nutritional Cleansing Program from Natural Factors that I codeveloped with Michael Lyon, M.D. This program comes in a boxed kit with a small booklet that contains detailed, easy-to-follow instructions on how to use the medicinal food powders and supplements in the kit as well as dietary guidelines, menu suggestions, and recipes. This is not a fast but a cleansing program designed to feed your body what it needs to get rid of the toxins. For more information on this program and where to get it, go to www.naturalfactors.com.

If you would rather use a "do it yourself" program, here is what I would recommend. Go on a three- to four-day fresh "juice fast" consisting of three or four 8-ounce juice meals spread throughout the day. Here are the guidelines:

- ▶ Although a short juice fast can be started at any time, it is best to begin on a weekend or at some other time when adequate rest can be ensured. The more rest, the better the results, as energy can be directed toward healing instead of other body functions.

- ▶ Only fresh fruit juices and vegetable juices (ideally prepared from organic produce) should be consumed for the next three to four days.

Four 8-ounce glasses of fresh juice should be consumed throughout the day. In addition to the fresh juice, pure water should also be liberally consumed. The quantity of water should be dictated by thirst, but at least four 8-ounce glasses should be consumed every day during the fast.

▸ Do not drink coffee; bottled, canned, or frozen juice; or soft drinks. Herbal teas can be quite supportive of a fast, but they should not be sweetened.

▸ Exercise is not usually encouraged during a fast. It is a good idea to conserve energy and allow maximal healing. Short walks or light stretching are useful, but heavy workouts tax the system and inhibit repair and elimination.

▸ Rest is one of the most important aspects of a fast. A nap or two during the day is recommended. Less sleep will usually be required at night, since daily activity is lower. Body temperature usually drops during a fast, as do blood pressure, pulse, and respiratory rate—all measures of the slowing of the metabolic rate of the body. It is important, therefore, to stay warm.

▸ Support your body's ability to detoxify by taking the following nutritional supplements:

  ▷ Take a high-potency multiple vitamin and mineral formula to provide general support.

  ▷ Take 500 to 1,000 (mg) of vitamin C three times daily.

  ▷ Take two capsules of Natural Factors' Liver Health Formula twice daily.

  ▷ Take 20 to 25 grams (g) of undenatured whey protein daily.

  ▷ Take 1 to 2 tablespoons of powdered psyllium seed husks, ReNew Life's Organic Triple Fiber, or Natural Factors' Enriching Greens.

Drink Water!

Low fluid consumption in general and low water consumption in particular make it difficult for the body to eliminate toxins. As a result, low water consumption increases the risk of cancer. Drinking enough water is another basic habit for good health, as you've probably heard 1,000 times. It's true: you need to drink at least six to eight glasses of water (48 to 64 ounces) each day. That means having a glass of water every two waking hours. Don't wait until you're thirsty; schedule regular water breaks throughout the day instead.

Water is essential for life. The average amount of water in your body is about 10 gallons. We need to drink at least 48 ounces of water per day to replace the water that is lost through urination, sweat, and breathing. If we don't, we are likely to become dehydrated.

Even mild dehydration results in impaired physiological and performance responses. Many nutrients dissolve in water so that they can be absorbed more easily in your digestive tract. Similarly, many metabolic processes need to take place in water. Water is a component of blood and thus is important for transporting chemicals and nutrients to cells and tissues. Each of your cells is constantly bathed in a watery fluid. Water also carries waste materials from cells to the kidneys so they can be filtered out and eliminated. Water absorbs and transports heat. For example, heat produced by muscle cells during exercise is carried by water in the blood to the surface, helping your body maintain the right temperature balance. The skin cells also release water as perspiration, which helps keep you cool.

Several factors are thought to increase the likelihood of chronic, mild dehydration: a faulty thirst "alarm" in the brain; dissatisfaction with the taste of water; regular exercise that increases the amount of water lost through sweat; living in a hot, dry climate; and consumption of the natural diuretics caffeine and alcohol. Diuretics are substances that draw water out of your cells and increase the rate of urination. Surprisingly, if you drink two cups of water and two cups of coffee, cola, or beer, you may end up with a net water intake of zero! Be aware of your "water budget." If you drink coffee or other dehydrating beverages, compensate by drinking an additional glass of water.

▶ When it is time to break your fast, it is important to reintroduce solid foods gradually by limiting portions. Do not overeat. It is also a good idea to eat slowly, chew thoroughly, and eat foods at room temperature.

A NEGATIVE ATTITUDE, ANGER, AND PESSIMISM ARE MAJOR OBSTACLES TO HEALING

A positive mental attitude is one of the important, fundamental elements of good health. This principle has been contemplated by philosophers and physicians since the time of Plato and Hippocrates, and it is also simple common sense. Modern research has verified the importance that attitude—the collection of habitual thoughts and emotions—plays in determining the length and quality of life. Specifically, studies using various scales to assess attitude have shown that compared with optimists, individuals with a pessimistic attitude have poorer health, are prone to depression, are more frequent users of medical and mental health care delivery systems, exhibit more cognitive decline and impaired immune function with aging, and have a shorter survival rate. This research highlights the fact that although life is full of events that are beyond one's control, people can control their responses to such events. Attitude goes a long way toward determining how people view and respond to the stresses and challenges of life.

TYPE A PERSONALITY AND THE EXPRESSION OF ANGER

Type A behavior is characterized by an extreme sense of time urgency, competitiveness, impatience, and aggressiveness. This behavior carries with it a twofold increase in coronary heart disease (CHD) compared with non–type A behavior. Particularly damaging to the cardiovascular system is the regular expression of anger. In fact, research has shown that traits like time urgency and competitiveness are not associated with early death, but negative emotions, anger, and aggressive expression of anger were all associated with an increased risk of a heart attack, and high levels of hostility increased the chance of dying early from other diseases (e.g., cancer) as well. Hence, it can be argued that anger and hostility are a major cause of premature death.[8, 9]

The mechanisms underlying the effects of anger on cardiovascular disease are being explored. In one study, the relationship between habitual anger, coping styles, especially expression of anger, and serum lipid concentrations were examined. Habitual expression of anger was measured on four scales: aggression, controlled affect, guilt, and social inhibition. The results showed that the higher the aggression score, the higher the cholesterol level. Conversely, the greater the ability to control anger, the lower the ratio of LDL to HDL. In other words, those who learn to control anger experience a significant reduction in the risk of heart disease, whereas an unfavorable lipid profile is linked to a predominantly aggressive (hostile) style of coping with anger.[10]

Expression of anger also fuels the underlying inflammation that contributes to atherosclerosis (hardening of the arteries) and other diseases, including cancer, Alzheimer's disease, and diabetes. Levels of C-reactive protein (CRP) are used as a marker for this sort of inflammation and have been shown to correlate more strongly than cholesterol levels with risk of a heart attack or stroke. In one study, greater anger and severity of depressive symptoms, separately and in combination with hostility, were significantly associated with elevations in CRP. Other mechanisms explaining the link between expression of anger and cardiovascular disease include increased secretion of stress hormones such as cortisol, dysfunction in the lining of the arteries, high blood pressure, and formation of blood clots.[11, 12]

The conclusion to be drawn from all of this research is that expression of hostility and anger comes back to cause harm to the individual expressing it, as well as harming the original victims. Here are 10 tips for improving your coping strategies and reducing your feelings of anger and hostility:

1. Do not starve your emotional life. Foster meaningful relationships. Provide time to give and receive love in your life.

2. Learn to be a good listener. Allow the people in your life to share their feelings and thoughts uninterrupted. Empathize with them; put yourself in their shoes.

3. Do not try to talk over somebody. If you find yourself being interrupted, relax; do not try to outtalk the other person. If you are courteous and allow others to speak, eventually (unless they are extremely rude) they will respond likewise. If not, explain that they are interrupting the communication process. You can do this only if you have been a good listener.

4. Avoid aggressive or passive behavior. Be assertive, but express your thoughts and feelings in a kind way to help improve relationships at work and at home.

5. Avoid excessive stress in your life as best you can by avoiding excessive work hours, poor nutrition, and inadequate rest. Get as much sleep as you can.

6. Avoid stimulants like caffeine and nicotine. Stimulants promote the fight-or-flight response and tend to make people more irritable.

7. Take time to build long-term health and success by performing stress-reduction techniques and deep breathing exercises.

8. Accept gracefully those things over which you have no control. Save your energy for those things that you can do something about.

9. Accept yourself. Remember that you are human and will make mistakes from which you can learn along the way.

10. Be more patient and tolerant of other people. Follow the Golden Rule.

FROM GRIZZLY BEAR TO TEDDY BEAR

My favorite example of the healing power of a merry heart is Jerry. At the time of his first visit he was a 52-year-old employee of the United States Postal Service, on leave because of a medical disability. In the 11 years since he'd turned 41, Jerry had undergone seven heart surgeries—three coronary artery bypass operations and four angioplasties. Despite all these procedures and all the drugs he was taking, Jerry had intense angina on even slight exertion. The first time that I saw him, in fact, he had an angina attack just walking the few feet from the waiting room to my office. He quickly popped a nitroglycerine pill; it was just one of 11 prescription drugs he was taking, some of which were designed to reduce the side effects of other drugs.

Jerry was suffering from a severe case of heart failure; these medications were necessary in order to keep his weakened heart beating well enough to keep him alive. Jerry's heart disease was so grave that he was on the waiting list for a heart transplant. An extremely fascinating feature in Jerry's case is that he had no risk factors identifiable by conventional testing. His cholesterol levels were perfect, his blood pressure was actually low, he did not smoke, and he was not overweight. For years, his doctors had been at a loss to explain why he had such serious heart disease.

It didn't take long for me to figure it out. Jerry seemed like a very affable, mild-mannered guy. But when I asked him how he would evaluate his ability to control his temper, I could see that he often "went postal." I found it ironic that he was a postal worker. He told me that he was a real hothead and that his temper was a major problem in his life. I once made the mistake of asking him to give me some examples of what made him mad. His face turned red, the veins in his neck and forehead popped out, and his voice became quite loud as he told me a few things that really ticked him off. Shortly into this tirade he stopped for a second or two to pop another nitroglycerin pill.

At that point, I seized the opportunity to help him make the connection between his inability to control his anger and his heart disease. He was quite resistant at first, because he just wanted me to prescribe some natural medicines. Although I did provide him with a supplement regimen, I knew that the real key to getting him better was for him to take a look at his emotional life. It did not happen all at once, but over the next few visits he really opened up and became receptive to my ideas. One of my initial prescriptions to Jerry was to read a book by a noted cardiologist, my friend Dr. Stephen Sinatra: *Heartbreak and Heart Disease*. It is an excellent account of the role emotions play in heart disease. I also referred Jerry to a psychotherapist for biofeedback training and to a yoga instructor so that he could start taking yoga classes.

Within two years after I first saw Jerry, he went from popping nitroglycerin tablets nearly every time he got up out of his chair to walking nearly four miles per day. His heart function went from less than 20 percent of normal, despite his being on so many drugs, to nearly 80 percent of normal without any prescription medicines at all. Even more impressive than the improvements in his physical health were the changes in his emotional health and personality. What impressed me most, in fact, was the change in Jerry's relationship with his wife and kids.

What led to the improvement? Was it the natural medicines I prescribed for Jerry, or the changes he made in his emotional responses? No doubt the natural medicines that I prescribed improved his physical well-being. But I am convinced that the most important factor in Jerry's remarkable case was the emotional change he made. By making this change Jerry eliminated the major obstacle to wellness in his life.

FINAL COMMENT

I guarantee you that every doctor has observed at least one patient overcome an apparently terminal illness or a seemingly hopeless condition and make a miraculously recovery. What factors cause these remarkable occurrences? My belief is that they often involve removal of obstacles to healing. When I was a third-year medical student at Bastyr University, I observed something almost unbelievable that has stuck with me all these years. The case involved Jim, a 38-year-old man with cataracts. Now, cataracts simply do not form in someone that young unless the patient has a rare metabolic disease, uncontrolled diabetes, or damage—none of which applied to this patient Jim. Well, when the supervising doctor came in to examine Jim and review our assessment and plan, my clinic partner and I focused on possible biochemical explanations for the cataracts and a treatment program designed to address these possible abnormalities. I was very fortunate that the supervising doctor, Farrah Swan, N.D., was so insightful. After respectfully listening to us, she asked Jim a truly remarkable question: "Are there things happening in your life that you would rather not see?" Jim's response was a catharsis. There were several sources of pain in his life that he was dealing with—a mother on her deathbed, an alcoholic father drinking himself to death, and painful childhood memories of physical and sexual abuse.

Dr. Swan went on to explain to us that there is often a link between the mind and the symptoms and illnesses that our bodies express. As physicians we can look at the body as a script that the mind is writing. In Jim's case, we referred him to our psychology clinic and his response was truly miraculous. Within three months his well-formed cataracts were no longer present. Most doctors will tell you that this sort of response is not possible, and that is exactly my point. The human body has an incredible ability to heal spontaneously when the obstacles to healing are removed.

4

FUNCTIONAL MEDICINE VERSUS THE TREATMENT OF DISEASE

"The part can never be well unless the whole is well."
—Plato

OF ALL NATURE'S MIRACLES, the human body is the most amazing. As Thoreau realized, nature works constantly to ensure that your body functions well. Health is our natural state. But the body is complex and intricate—a collection of interweaving systems, each dependent on the others. Although we sometimes talk about the "parts" of our bodies, we are closer to the truth when we think of the body as a whole. At each moment, the body tries to maintain an ideal internal state. The technical term for this process is "homeostasis," which means "same standing." Every organism on the planet, from the simplest single-celled amoeba to the human being, relies on this internal mechanism, homeostasis, to sustain life.

Often, though, we subject our bodies to severe stress. If the homeostatic mechanism cannot overcome the forces that threaten it, then the system falls out of balance. In the worst cases, it fails completely. The result is disease ("dis-ease")—a disruption in the ability of a body system or part to carry out its normal function. By keeping our systems in tune, we can protect ourselves against disease and enjoy the benefits of health.

No matter how old you are or what your current state of health is, you can take steps to help your body function better. You can work better, feel better, and look better—all by taking some basic steps to help your body maintain its optimal homeostasis.

In my years of practice, I found that most of my patients are very good at knowing when something isn't quite right with their body. But often they feel discouraged because they have visited doctors who tell them that there is nothing wrong. Often, this means that their doctors have been unable to diagnose a specific disease, something that can be looked up in their textbooks or pointed to under a microscope. My perspective is different. I practice what is called *functional medicine*, an approach pioneered by the nutritional biochemist Jeffrey Bland, Ph.D. In functional medicine, the presence or absence of a disease is secondary to an understanding of the function that prevents a disease or the dysfunction that allows a disease to occur.

A significant difference in the functional approach to health versus the disease-centered approach is that often a body system or an organ can be functioning poorly but be free of disease per se. In these situations, conventional medicine has little to offer to improve the function. Sometimes, a simple correction of diet, proper supplementation, or some lifestyle change can produce dramatic improvements in symptoms more effectively than drugs. Moreover, when prescription or over-the-counter drugs are used to try to suppress the symptoms in a case where no disease process is occurring, they tend to produce side effects and sometimes these side effects can be life-threatening. To illustrate the difference in the approaches, there are many examples to choose from. Perhaps the best examples are simple disorders of digestion.

THE IRRATIONAL APPROACH TO INDIGESTION

The term "indigestion" is often used by patients to describe heartburn, upper abdominal pain, a feeling of gaseousness, difficulty swallowing, a feeling of pressure or heaviness after eating, a sensation of bloating after eating, stomach or abdominal pains and cramps, or fullness in the abdomen. The medical terms used to describe indigestion include functional dyspepsia (FD), non-ulcer dyspepsia (NUD), and gastroesophageal reflux disease (GERD).

These are among the most common diagnoses in North America, and yet several review articles have concluded that "the efficacy of current drugs on the market is limited at best." "At best" signifies that often these drugs cause more problems than they solve.

Various drugs are used in the treatment of indigestion, FD, NUD, GERD, and irritable bowel syndrome (IBS). My point here is not to show you how ludicrous all these drugs are as a treatment for such functional disorders. Instead, I want to focus on the most popular—acid-blocking drugs. These drugs work, as the term implies, by blocking one of the most important digestive processes, the secretion of hydrochloric acid by the stomach.

Acid-blocker drugs are divided into two general groups. One group consists of the older histamine-receptor antagonist drugs, including Zantac, Tagamet, and Pepcid AC. The other consists of newer and more potent drugs called proton-pump inhibitors (PPIs), including Nexium, Prilosec, Protonix, Prevacid, and Aciphex.

These drugs are a huge business; their total prescription and over-the-counter (OTC) sales are estimated to exceed $13 billion annually. The drug companies love them because they are expensive, don't produce a true cure, but do tend to suppress symptoms. In short, when people start taking one of these drugs they tend to become dependent on it, and for good reason—it interferes with the body's natural digestive processes and produces significant disturbances in the gastrointestinal tract. Also, these drugs are typically quite expensive; and as my colleague Jacob Schor, N.D., has noted, "New research on their side effects says that the money spent on acid blocking drugs may be the least of the costs of using them."

Acid-blocking drugs will typically raise the gastric pH above the normal range of 3.5, effectively inhibiting the action of pepsin, an enzyme involved in protein digestion that can be irritating to the stomach. Although raising the pH can reduce symptoms, it also substantially blocks a normal body process. The production and secretion of stomach acid are very important not only to the digestive process but also as a protective mechanism against infection. Stomach secretions can neutralize bacteria, viruses, and molds before these can cause gastrointestinal infection. With regard to the digestive process, stomach acid helps initiate protein digestion and it ionizes minerals and other nutrients for enhanced absorption; and without sufficient secretion of hydrochloric acid (HCl) in the stomach the pancreas does not get the signal to secrete its digestive enzymes.

Background of the New Purple Pill

One of the most expensive marketing campaigns in the history of the drug industry was the nearly $500 million spent by AstraZeneca to switch people from its profitable drug Prilosec to the "new purple pill" Nexium. In 2000, Prilosec was the world's largest-selling prescription drug, with annual sales of more than $6 billion, and it accounted for 39 percent of AstraZeneca's income. The problem for AstraZeneca was that the patent protection for Prilosec was due to expire in 2001. The loss of patent protection would mean the introduction of generic versions that would be priced significantly lower.

Fortunately for Astra-Zeneca, just before the patent was about to expire, it received FDA approval for Nexium. To protect its profits, AstraZeneca began the $500 million campaign with ads appearing everywhere proclaiming, "Today's purple pill is Nexium, from the makers of Prilosec." The company also added 1,300 sales reps to promote the product directly to physicians. As a result, the introduction and promotion of Nexium allowed AstraZeneca to prevent the revenue loss it would have experienced with competition from generics. In 2003, although revenues from Prilosec slid to under $1 billion as many patients and doctors switched to less expensive generic alternatives, sales of Nexium were $3.9 billion. Even when Prilosec did go OTC in 2004, AstraZeneca managed, by "accidental" shortages of the identical OTC version, to keep up sales of the prescription version, which costs six times as much.

Is Nexium better than Prilosec? Here the story gets even more interesting. Chemically, Nexium contains the left-handed version whereas while Prilosec contains both the left- and the right-handed version of the same molecule (omeprazole). There is no real evidence that Nexium is any better, though AstraZeneca seemed to pull the wool over many doctors' eyes with some cleverly designed clinical trials. Rather than test Nexium versus Prilosec at equivalent dosages, the studies used by AstraZeneca to promote Nexium involved giving subjects with GERD a dosage 40 milligrams (mg) of Nexium but only 20 mg of Prilosec.[1, 2] Of course Nexium performed better. Since another study of patients with GERD showed that 20 mg of Prilosec was equal to 20 mg of Nexium,[3] there doesn't seem to be any real difference between the two other than the cost. Substituting OTC Prilosec for Nexium, Prevacid, and other prescription acid-blockers would cut spending on those medicines by about 50 percent, or almost $7 billion nationally—enough money to pay for health coverage for more than 1 million uninsured Americans— according to a study by the University of Arkansas.[4]

THE BACTERIAL LINK TO PEPTIC ULCER DISEASE

A corkscrew-shaped bacterium, *Helicobacter pylori* (*H. pylori*) is now regarded as the most important factor in the development of peptic ulcers and stomach cancer. The bacterium—one of the few that manage to survive in the acidic environment of the upper digestive tract—seems to burrow under the surface of the stomach lining and attach itself to the underlying cells. There it disrupts the production of the thick protective mucin lining the stomach and intestines and triggers localized inflammation that ultimately leads to the formation of ulcers.

In 2005, Barry Marshall and Robin Warren were awarded the Nobel Prize in Physiology or Medicine for their discovery, in 1979, that *H. pylori* is a primary factor in peptic ulcer disease and for their subsequent work. As a result, when doctors suspect that peptic ulcer is associated with *H. pylori* and is not due to other factors (such as side effects of drugs), they typically consider it an infection and treat it with antibiotics.

My take on this H. pylori link is that it is another instance in which conventional medicine is obsessed with an infective agent rather than focusing on the host's defense factors. Here is an analogy: Where there is garbage, there are likely to be flies. You can spray the garbage with insect repellent and control the flies for a little while, but if you take care of the garbage the flies will disappear permanently. The popular treatment of peptic ulcers is antibiotic therapy plus an acid-blocking drug, but the antibiotics are like insect repellent, and taking them in combination with an acid-blocking drug may be extremely dangerous (discussed below). A more rational approach is to focus on eliminating the factors that lead to an overgrowth of *H. pylori*. Unfortunately, because research focuses on killing the bacteria rather than increasing the health of the intestinal lining, there is little information on factors that protect against *H. pylori*. Proposed protective factors include maintaining a low pH through proper secretion of stomach acids. But that proposal raises a question: do acid-blocking drugs lead to ulcers? Most experts now agree that they do, because they promote the growth of *H. pylori*. As a result, the use of acid-blockers as the dominant medical treatment for peptic ulcers for more than 30 years is a classic example of a drug that effectively suppresses symptoms while simultaneously increasing the disease process.

IS TRIPLE THERAPY TRIPLE THE DANGER?

The standard first-line therapy for peptic ulcer now consists of taking an acid-blocking drug along with two antibiotics—amoxicillin and clarithromycin—for ten to fourteen days. It is known as "triple therapy" and is often quite effective in healing peptic ulcers, but it does pose significant risks, and an increasing number of people harbor antibiotic-resistant strains of *H. pylori*. As a result, the initial treatment fails and the infection requires additional rounds of antibiotic therapy or even stronger measures.

The risks are numerous, but they can be largely prevented with appropriate supplementation (discussed below). The acid-blocking drug removes an important barrier to infection, and the antibiotics kill off the health-promoting bacteria that line the intestines and normally protect the body from infecting organisms. To illustrate this potentially serious combination, researchers gave mice two kinds of live, antibiotic-resistant bacteria for three days. Then they gave the mice a very strong antibiotic (clindamycin) alone or in combination with Protonix, an acid-blocking drug. The results demonstrated that when mice were given both the acid-blocker drug and the antibiotic the infection rate was 75 to 85 percent; this was three times higher than the rate among mice given just the antibiotic.[5]

This study and many others are showing the importance of maintaining stomach pH and a normal gastrointestinal flora as barriers to infection. One of the major complications of using antibiotics is diarrhea caused by altering the type of bacteria in the colon or by promoting the overgrowth of *Candida albicans*. One of the most severe forms of antibiotic-induced diarrhea is pseudomembranous enterocolitis (PME). This condition is attributed to an overgrowth of a bacterium *(Clostridium difficele)*, resulting from the death of the bacteria that normally keep this *Clostridium* under control. Pseudomembranous enterocolitis can be quite serious and even deadly.

The risk of PME seems to be greatly increased if antibiotics are given in combination with acid-blocking drugs. In 1994, prior to the widespread use of the strong acid-blockers like Prilosec and Nexium, only one person in 100,000 developed PME. By 2004, the occurrence rate had jumped to 22 in 100,000. According to a report published in the *Journal of the American Medical Association* (JAMA), people who take proton-pump inhibitor acid-blocking drugs are three times more likely to develop PME than people not taking these drugs.[6] This figure is identical to the increase in infection rate shown in the study with mice.

PROTECTING YOURSELF FROM PME

Probiotics are friendly microflora (bacteria and other organisms) that are vital to our health. Probiotic products include free-dried bacteria available in capsules at health food stores, and also fermented foods such as yogurt, sauerkraut, and kefir. The specific microorganisms found in these products are usually lactobacilli and bifidobacteria species. These bacteria are the major probiotics in the human intestinal tract.

Anytime that you need to take an antibiotic or an acid-blocking drug it is vitally important to supplement your diet with probiotics. This recommendation is especially important if you are undergoing major surgery. Just prior to and after major surgery you will be given antibiotics to reduce the likelihood of an infection. That is very important, but without probiotic supplementation you run the risk of developing not only PME but other gastrointestinal infections as well.

Numerous clinical studies have shown that probiotic supplements produce good results in preventing and treating antibiotic-induced diarrhea.[7, 8, 9] Yet, this is an underutilized therapy even though it can prevent significant suffering and even death. Although probiotic supplements are commonly believed ineffective if taken during antibiotic therapy, research actually supports the use of probiotics during such therapy.

Here is something else most doctors don't know: a detailed analysis of several clinical trials showed that when probiotic supplements are used in a program to eradicate *H. pylori*, not only is there a reduction in side effects but the eradication rates also improve significantly.[10]

PRACTICAL RECOMMENDATIONS FOR USING PROBIOTIC SUPPLEMENTS

The intestinal flora plays a major role in the health of the host. Therefore, probiotic supplements can be used to promote overall good health. There are also numerous specific uses for probiotics, based on clinical studies.[7]

Promotion of proper intestinal environment

Stimulation of gastrointestinal tract and systemic immunity

Prevention and treatment of:

Antibiotic-induced diarrhea

Urinary tract infection

Vaginal yeast infections and bacterial vaginosis

Eczema

Food allergies

Cancer

Irritable bowel syndrome

Inflammatory bowel disease (ulcerative colitis, Crohn's disease)

Traveler's diarrhea

Lactose intolerance

Numerous analyses of commercially available probiotic supplements indicate that there is a tremendous range of quality. The quality of probiotic supplements depends on two main factors: (1) the characteristics of the strains contained in the supplement and (2) adequate viability, so that sufficient numbers of bacteria are viable at the point of consumption. Viability at consumption depends on a number of factors, such as proper manufacturing and the hardiness of the strain, as well as packaging and storage of the product in the right amount of moisture and at the correct temperature.

Strains of bacteria can be likened to breeds of dogs. All dogs belong to the genus *Canis* and the species *familiaris*. Within this one species is great diversity in size, shape, strength, and other physical characteristics—breeds range from the Saint Bernard to the Chihuahua. A similar division occurs within species of bacteria. Within each species of bacteria there is a multitude of strains. Some probiotic strains are resilient and strong, able to survive passage through the upper gastrointestinal tract and inhibit pathogenic bacteria; others are weak and cannot survive or kill pathogenic bacteria.

Therefore, consumers must utilize products developed and manufactured by companies that have done the necessary research to ensure the viability of their product. There are some very good companies offering high-quality probiotic supplements, but there are also some companies selling products that do not come anywhere close to the claims on the labels. Obviously, the product that I recommend over all others is the one that I developed—Ultimate Probiotic from Natural Factors. But there are many other high-quality probiotic supplements, including Healthy Trinity from Natren, Culturelle® with Lactobacillus GG, and Nature's Way Primadophilus Optima.

The dosage of probiotic supplements is based solely on the number of live organisms present in the product; therefore, I recommend using products that list the number of live bacteria at expiration rather than at time of manufacture. Successful results are most often attained by taking between 5 billion and 20 billion viable bacteria per day.

BISMUTH—UNDERAPPRECIATED AND UNDERUTILIZED IN ELIMINATING *H. PYLORI*

Bismuth is a naturally occurring mineral that can act as an antacid as well as against *H. pylori*. Bismuth preparations are now often prescribed along with triple therapy as a component in quadruple therapy for the eradication of *H. pylori*. The best-known and most widely used bismuth preparation is bismuth subsalicylate (Pepto-Bismol). However, bismuth subcitrate has produced the best results against *H. pylori* and in the treatment of non-ulcer-related indigestion as well as peptic ulcers.[11] In the United States, bismuth subcitrate preparations are available by prescription through compounding pharmacies (contact the International Academy of Compounding Pharmacists, www.iacprx.org, 1-800-927-4227).

One of the main advantages of bismuth preparations over standard antibiotic approaches to eradicating *H. pylori* is that whereas the bacteria may develop resistance to various antibiotics, they are very unlikely to develop resistance to bismuth.

The usual dosage for bismuth subcitrate is 240 milligrams (mg) twice daily before meals. For bismuth subsalycilate the dosage is 500 mg—two tablets or 30 milliliters (mL) of standard-strength Pepto-Bismol—four times daily.

Bismuth preparations are extremely safe when taken at prescribed dosages and for less than six weeks at a time. Bismuth subcitrate may cause a temporary and harmless darkening of the tongue, the stool, or both. Bismuth subsalicylate should not be taken by children recovering from the flu, chicken pox, or some other viral infections, as it may mask the nausea and vomiting associated with Reye's syndrome, a rare but serious illness.

OTHER SIDE EFFECTS OF
ACID-BLOCKING DRUGS

As a class, these drugs are associated with numerous side effects, but they are for some reason generally regarded as safe and many are now available over the counter. However, because these drugs block a vital bodily function involved in digestion, digestive disturbances are quite common and can include nausea, constipation, and diarrhea. Nutrient deficiencies can appear as a result of impaired digestion. Other possible side effects include allergic reactions, headaches, breast enlargement in men (with Tagamet and Zantac), hair loss, and dizziness. Here are some additional concerns about acid-blockers that you typically will not find on patient handouts from a pharmacy.

▶ Pneumonia—People using acid-blockers were 4.5 times as likely to develop pneumonia as people who never used these drugs. Apparently, without acid in the stomach bacteria from the intestine can migrate upstream to reach the throat and then the lungs to cause infection.[12]

▶ Increased fractures—People taking high doses of proton-pump inhibitors (PPIs) for longer than a year had a 260 percent increase in rates of hip fractures compared with people not taking an acid-blocker. Evidence suggests that PPIs may disrupt bone remodeling, making bones weaker and more susceptible to fracture.[13]

▶ Vitamin B_{12} insufficiency—Acid-blocking drugs reduce the secretion not only of stomach acid but also of intrinsic factor (a compound that binds to and assists the absorption of vitamin B_{12}).[14] Vitamin B_{12} deficiency is among the most common nutritional deficiencies in older people. Depending on the testing method used, studies indicate that 10 to 43 percent of the elderly are deficient in vitamin B_{12} and are consequently at risk of several health problems, including dementia. Many elderly people who are placed in nursing homes for Alzheimer's disease may simply be suffering from vitamin B_{12} deficiency.

WHAT ABOUT ANTACIDS?

Over-the-counter antacids are usually safe and effective when taken occasionally to relieve heartburn, but some important distinctions need to be made:

▸ *Be careful not to abuse antacids.* Regular use can lead to such side effects as malabsorption of nutrients, bowel irregularities, and kidney stones. Furthermore, although antacids often provide immediate relief, they can produce what is known as acid rebound three or four hours after use. This means that the body will try to overcompensate for the neutralization of gastric acid by secreting even more acid. While this may not be a problem in treating indigestion, it may play a role in delaying the healing of ulcers.

▸ *Limit the use of sodium bicarbonate.* Many people take sodium bicarbonate (baking soda) for relief of acid indigestion. (Alka-Seltzer is simply ordinary baking soda in a fizzy form.) Although sodium bicarbonate can be useful in the short term, using it often or regularly can increase your sodium intake to unnecessarily high levels. Long-term administration can cause systemic alkalosis (excessively high pH levels throughout the body), leading to such complications as the formation of kidney stones, nausea, vomiting, headache, and mental confusion.

▸ *Avoid antacids that contain aluminum.* These products (such as Maalox, Rolaids, Digel, Mylanta, and Riopan) have issues of long-term safety due to the aluminum in them. Aluminum may play a role in impairing mental function as well as in diseases of the nervous system including Alzheimer's disease, Parkinson's disease, and Lou Gehrig's disease (amyotrophic lateral sclerosis). Absorption of aluminum is made worse if a meal contains any source of citric acid, such as citrus fruit, juice, or soda pop. In my opinion, there is no reason to use aluminum-containing antacids, because the potential risks far outweigh the short-term benefit.

▶ *Follow dosage instructions.* It is especially important to avoid taking too much of a magnesium salt such as magnesium oxide, hydroxide, or carbonate. Besides acting as a mild antacid, magnesium salts can exert a laxative effect making diarrhea a definite risk.

THE NATURAL APPROACH TO TREATING INDIGESTION

For a person with chronic indigestion, rather than focusing on blocking the digestive process with antacids, the rational approach is to focus on aiding digestion. Indigestion can be attributed to a great many causes, including not only increased secretion of acid but also decreased secretion of acid and other digestive factors and enzymes. In fact, most nutrition-oriented physicians believe that lack of acid, not an excess, is the true culprit in many patients with indigestion.

The first step is eliminating common dietary causes of GERD and NUD. These causes include overeating, coffee, chocolate, fried foods, carbonated beverages (soft drinks), and alcohol. Another cause is obesity. In many cases, simply eliminating or reducing causative foods or beverages is all that is necessary to completely relieve GERD or NUD. Other tips include decreasing the size of portions at mealtime; chewing food thoroughly; eating in a leisurely manner in a calm, relaxed atmosphere; and not eating within two hours of bedtime.

A number of natural products that can be very effective in relieving GERD and NUD. Although much is said about hyperacidity, a more common cause of indigestion is insufficient secretion of gastric acid. Hypochlorhydria is deficient secretion of gastric acid and achlorhydria is a complete absence of such secretion. Like peptic ulcer disease, achlorhydria and hypochlorhydria have been linked to overgrowth of *H. pylori*.

Many symptoms and signs suggest impaired secretion of gastric acid, and a number of specific diseases have been found to be associated with insufficient output of gastric acid.

Common Signs and Symptoms of Low Gastric Acidity

Bloating, belching, burning, and flatulence immediately after meals

Sense of fullness after eating

Indigestion, diarrhea, or constipation

Multiple food allergies

Nausea after taking supplements

Itching around the rectum

Weak, peeling, cracked fingernails

Dilated blood vessels in the cheeks and nose

Acne

Iron deficiency

Chronic intestinal parasites or abnormal flora

Undigested food in stool

Chronic candida infections

Gassiness in the upper digestive tract

Diseases Associated with Low Gastric Acidity

Addison's disease

Asthma

Celiac disease

Dermatitis herpetiformis

Diabetes mellitus

Eczema

Gallbladder disease

Graves disease

Chronic autoimmune disorders

Hepatitis

Chronic hives

Lupus erythematosis

Myasthenia gravis

Osteoporosis

Pernicious anemia

Psoriasis

Rheumatoid arthritis

Rosacea

Sjogren's syndrome

Thyrotoxicosis

Hyper- and hypothyroidism

Vitiligo

Since not everyone can have detailed gastric acid analysis to determine the need for supplementation, let me offer a practical method of determination to use if you are experiencing any signs and symptoms of gastric acid insufficiency:

▸ Begin by taking one tablet or capsule containing 10 grains (600 mg) of hydrochloric acid (HCl) at your next large meal. If this does not aggravate your symptoms, at every subsequent meal of the same size take one more tablet or capsule. (Two at the next meal, three at the meal after that, then four at the next meal.)

▶ Continue to increase the dose until you reach seven tablets, or when you feel warmth in your stomach, whichever occurs first. A feeling of warmth in the stomach means that you have taken too many tablets for the meal, and you need to take one less tablet for a meal of that size. It is a good idea to try the larger dose again at another meal to make sure that it was the HCl that caused the warmth and not something else.

▶ After you have found the largest dose that you can take at your large meals without feeling any warmth, maintain that dose at all meals of similar size. You will need to take fewer tablets or capsules at smaller meals.

▶ When you take a number of tablets or capsules, it is best to take them throughout the meal.

▶ As your stomach begins to regain the ability to produce the amount of HCl needed to properly digest your food, you will notice the warm feeling again and will have to cut down the dosage.

DIGESTIVE ENZYMES

Lack of digestive enzymes from the pancreas is another functional cause of indigestion. Typically when heartburn, abdominal bloating, abdominal discomfort, and gas occur within the first 15 to 30 minutes after eating, the cause is usually a lack of HCl secretion. If these effects occur after 45 minutes, they usually indicate a lack of pancreatic enzymes. Keep in mind that the secretion of pancreatic enzymes is triggered by the HCl secreted in the stomach. So sometimes taking HCl supplements can lead to improved release of pancreatic enzymes.

Digestive enzyme products are the most effective treatment for pancreatic insufficiency. These preparations can include enzymes from fresh hog pancreas (pancreatin) or vegetarian sources, such as bromelain and papain (protein-digesting enzymes from pineapple and papaya, respectively); and fungal enzymes. I have found that the best results are obtained with multi-enzyme preparations derived from vegetarian sources. They are definitely more resistant to digestive secretions and have a broader range of activity. Simply follow the label instructions for the proper dosage.

A NATURAL CURE FOR PEPTIC ULCERS AND GERD

My all-time favorite natural medicine is a special extract of licorice root known as DGL. (It is short for deglycyrrhizinated licorice, but I tell my patients that it stands for "darn good licorice.") It is produced by removing glycyrrhetinic acid—a compound that can cause elevations in blood pressure due to sodium and water retention. (Yes, eating too much licorice candy can raise blood pressure.) Because the glycyrrhetinic acid has been removed, DGL does not raise blood pressure.

My fondness for DGL is a result of having used it effectively to treat even the most severe peptic ulcers as well as to relieve the symptoms associated with GERD. In fact, I cannot think of a case in which DGL did not work. Rather than inhibit the release of acid, DGL stimulates the normal defense mechanisms that prevent ulcers. It improves both the quality and the quantity of the protective substances that line the intestinal tract, increases the life span of the intestinal cell, and improves blood supply to the intestinal lining. There is also some evidence that it inhibits the growth of *H. pylori*.[15]

Several clinical studies published over the years support my experience. In head-to-head studies, DGL has been shown to be more effective than Tagamet, Zantac, or antacids in both short-term treatment and maintenance therapy for peptic ulcers.[16, 17]

The standard dosage for DGL is two to four 380-mg chewable tablets taken between meals or twenty minutes before meals. Taking DGL after meals or taking it in a non-chewable form is associated with poor results. The DGL therapy should be continued for at least eight to 16 weeks after there is a full therapeutic response.

PEPPERMINT OIL FOR GERD, NUD, AND IBS

Peppermint oil placed in special capsules that are coated (enteric-coated) to prevent their breakdown in the stomach has been shown to be quite helpful in improving gastrointestinal function in individuals with irritable bowel syndrome (IBS). This is a common functional disorder of the large intestine characterized by some combination of the following: (1) abdominal pain; (2) altered bowel function, constipation, or diarrhea; (3) hypersecretion of colonic mucus; (4) dyspeptic symptoms (flatulence, nausea, anorexia); and (5) varying degrees of anxiety or depression.

In several double-blind studies, enteric-coated peppermint oil (ECPO) has been shown to be effective in relieving all symptoms of IBS in approximately 70 to 85 percent of cases within a two to four weeks. In addition, ECPO has benefits in treating NUD and GERD, and in eradicating *H. pylori*.[18]

Several clinical studies of patients with IBS used a combination of peppermint oil and caraway oil. The results of these trials indicate that this combination produces better results than peppermint oil alone for symptoms of IBS. Recent studies also indicate the combination of peppermint and caraway oil is more helpful in improving NUD. In one double-blind study, 120 patients with NUD were given either the peppermint and caraway seed oil (ECPO) or cisapride (Propulsid) for four weeks.[19] Symptoms of NUD, including pain, were reduced equally in both groups. Positive results were also found in *H. pylori*–positive individuals.

The significance of this study is enormous. Whereas enteric-coated peppermint and caraway oil is extremely safe at recommended levels, Propulsid was linked to fatal problems with heart rhythm. Once a popular medication for GERD and NUD marketed by Johnson and Johnson, Propulsid was pulled from the market in July 2000 after being linked to 341 reports of abnormalities in heart rhythm. According to the FDA, at least 111 people died as a result of using Propulsid, and nearly 400 developed heart abnormalities. A particularly alarming fact, which came to light after Propulsid was pulled, is that in one study of 58,000 premature babies' medical records, 20 percent of the babies were found to have been given Propulsid.

The usual dosage of enteric-coated capsules containing peppermint and caraway seed oil is one or two 200-mg capsules up to three times daily between meals. Side effects are rare, but can include allergic reactions (skin rash), heartburn, and—if the dosage is too high—a burning sensation on defecation. There are no known drug interactions.

FINAL COMMENTS

One of the most common digestive issues is constipation, which now affects more than 4 million Americans. The primary reason is lack of dietary fiber. In addition, some people develop unhealthy habits that actually "train" the bowel to become constipated. For example, they ignore the "call of nature" and do not use the toilet as soon as the urge strikes. Other people become dependent on laxatives to produce a bowel movement. Fortunately, it is possible to retrain your body and develop a more regular pattern of bowel movements.

- ► Eat a high-fiber diet, particularly fruits and vegetables.

- ► Drink six to eight glasses of fluids per day.

- ► Identify known causes of constipation, such as not enough fiber in the diet or the use of drugs like diuretics.

- ► Do not repress an urge to defecate; use the toilet as soon as you can.

- ► Sit on the toilet at the same time every day (even when the urge to defecate is not present), preferably immediately after breakfast or exercise.

- ► Exercise at least twenty minutes, three times per week.

- ► Take 3 to 5 grams (g) of a gel-forming fiber supplement (e.g., Metamucil and other psyllium preparations are fine) at night before retiring.

For children with a history of constipation, the first thing I recommend is eliminating milk and other dairy products from the diet. It is well accepted that intolerance to cow's milk (either an allergy or lactose intolerance) can produce diarrhea. What is not as well known is the fact that cow's milk intolerance can also lead to constipation and is a major cause of childhood constipation.[20] About 70 percent of cases of childhood constipation are cured by eliminating cow's milk from the diet and substituting soy or rice milk. Kids with constipation who respond to the elimination of milk also experience a decreased symptoms of allergy, including runny nose, eczema, and asthma. My recommendation is that if your child is constipated, start by eliminating cow's milk and other dairy products while increasing the intake of high-fiber foods, especially pears, apples, and other whole fruits. If this approach is not successful, try barley malt extract available at any health food store. Avoid mineral oil and stimulant laxatives unless they are absolutely necessary.

5

IS SYMPTOM RELIEF A
PATH TO BAD MEDICINE?

"A headache is not caused by a deficiency of aspirin."
—William Mitchell, N.D., cofounder of Bastyr University

THE HISTORY OF CONVENTIONAL medicine illustrates quite clearly how a treatment that is in vogue at a particular time can later be viewed as completely irrational and counterproductive. Were the physicians of the late nineteenth century as convinced of the efficacy of the dominant treatments of the time (such as bloodletting and the use of toxic compounds, including mercury) as today's physicians are about their treatments? Undoubtedly, and sadly, the answer is often yes. Certainly there are many safe and effective medical treatments, but I do believe there is a fundamental flaw in the use of most drugs: conventional drugs rarely have a curative effect. Instead they simply act as biochemical Band-Aids to make us feel better.

This focus on relieving symptoms often comes at a very high price. There are countless examples of drugs that take care of a primary symptom but have significant adverse consequences because they do not address the underlying cause. Some drugs create dependency; others interfere with normal physiology in a way that actually intensifies the very condition being treated; some produce side effects worse than the original symptoms.

CASE IN POINT: THE ALLOPATHIC
APPROACH TO A HEADACHE

To illustrate the problem that arises when we focus on suppressing symptoms rather than on determining causes, let's take a look at something very simple—a headache. Although a headache may be associated with a serious medical condition, most headaches are not serious. Headaches can be caused by a wide variety of factors, but the overwhelming majority are either tension or migraine headaches. A quick way to differentiate between the two is the nature of the pain. A tension headache is usually a steady, constant, dull pain that starts at the back of the head or in the forehead and spreads over the entire head, giving a sensation of pressure of a vise being applied to the skull. In contrast, migraine headaches are vascular headaches characterized by a throbbing or pounding sharp pain.

Modern drug treatment of the headache, whether a migraine or tension, is ultimately doomed because it fails to address the underlying cause, and as a result produces a significant risk of side effects. The goal of headache medications is not to identify and eliminate the precipitating factor, but simply to relieve the symptoms. Very interestingly, several clinical studies have estimated that in approximately 70 percent of patients with chronic daily headaches, the headaches are drug-induced. That is, their headaches are due to the medications they are taking to suppress the symptoms of a headache.[1] In other words, the headache medications are giving these patients daily headaches; and if they quit taking the drugs, their headaches go away. In one study (summarized below) of 200 patients suffering from analgesic rebound headache, discontinuation of these symptomatic medications resulted in 52 percent improvement in the total headache index. There were specific improvements in general well-being and sleep patterns, and a reduction in irritability, depression, lethargy, and the frequency and severity of headaches.

Profile of 200 Patients with Chronic Daily Headaches[1]

Medications	Average Number of Tablets per Week	Range of Number of Tablets per Week	Number of Patients	Percent of Patients
Butalbital/aspirin, acetaminophen/caffeine with or without codeine	30	14 to 86	84	42
Codeine	28	10 to 84	80	40
Aspirin or acetaminophen with caffeine	42	14 to 108	50	25
Ergotamine	15	6 to 42	44	22
Acetaminophen	52	15 to 105	34	17
Propxyphene	26	14 to 56	32	16
Nasal decongestants and antihistamines	14	6 to 30	24	12
Aspirin	28	10 to 64	8	4

WHAT CAUSES A TENSION HEADACHE?

If a tension headache is not caused by a deficiency of aspirin or acetamino-phen, then what does cause it? Well, there is a reason why it is called a ten-sion headache: it is usually caused by tightening in the muscles of the face, neck, or scalp as a result of stress or poor posture. The tightening of the muscles results in a pinching of a nerve or its blood supply, which in turn results in pain and pressure. Relaxation of the muscle usually brings imme-diate relief.

TREATING THE CAUSE OF TENSION HEADACHES

The primary therapy should address the factors that cause tension in the neck, face, or scalp muscles. Since the neck is an area of the body that often holds tension produced by psychological stress, it is especially important to learn techniques such as progressive relaxation (see page 35). In addition, it is important to address any structural factor that may be causing tension headaches. In particular, chiropractic can be quite helpful when misalignment of the spine creates muscular tension in the neck. Several clinical studies provide significant scientific evidence that chiropractic can provide benefits for many patients with neck pain and headaches.[2, 3, 4, 5] It is certainly worth a try. An alternative to chiropractic is getting a referral to a conventional physical therapist (PT) from your primary care doctor. Clinical studies have shown that conventional physical therapy consisting of education for posture at home and in the workplace, home exercise, massage, and

---

Relaxation Exercises Help Children with Chronic Headaches

Learning how to relax and diffuse tension goes a very long way in the treatment and prevention of tension headaches. Teaching people with chronic tension headaches how to relax, or using biofeedback therapies, has been shown, in clinical studies, to provide exceptional benefits without side effects. One of the more interesting studies considered the effectiveness of school-based relaxation training by nurses as a treatment for chronic tension headache in children (10–15 years old).[6] These children's headaches were, significantly reduced, compared with those of children in a no-treatment control group, after six weeks and at a six-month follow-up. At the time of the two evaluations, 69 percent and 73 percent of the students, respectively, trained in relaxation had achieved a clinically significant improvement (at least a 50 percent improvement) as compared with 8 percent and 27 percent of the children, respectively, in the no-treatment control group. The conclusion is that teaching kids with chronic tension headaches how to relax can be quite effective and is without side effects. What I really like about this therapy is that it sends kids a better message—rather than getting relief from a pill (drug), they learn how to control the headache themselves. This therapy was developed in Norway, and by now at least seven double-blind studies over a 20-year period support its effectiveness not only for tension headaches but also for migraines.[7]

stretching the cervical spine muscles can reduce the frequency and severity of tension headaches.

WHAT CAUSES A MIGRAINE HEADACHE?

Considerable evidence supports an association between migraine headaches and instability of blood vessels. The mechanism of migraine can be described as a three-stage process: (1) initiation, (2) prodrome (time between initiation and appearance of headache), and (3) headache. Although a particular trigger may be associated with the onset of a specific attack, it appears that initiation depends on an accumulation of several triggers over time. Once a critical point of susceptibility (or threshold) is reached, a "cascade event" is initiated, setting in process a domino effect that ultimately produces a headache. Food allergies, histamine-releasing foods, alcohol (especially red wine), stress, hormonal changes (e.g., menstruation, ovulation, birth control pills), and changes in weather (especially changes in barometric pressure) are some common triggers of migraines.

TREATING THE CAUSE OF A
MIGRAINE HEADACHE

The first step in treating a migraine headache is identifying the precipitating factor. Although food intolerance and allergy are most important, many other factors must be considered as either primary causes or contributors. In particular, it is important to assess the possible role of headache medications, especially in chronic headaches. Learning to deal with stress and learning how to relax are also critical. Just as in tension headaches, biofeedback and relaxation training can also be helpful. The effectiveness of biofeedback and relaxation training in reducing the frequency and severity of recurrent migraine headaches has been the subject of more than 35 clinical studies.[8, 9] When the results of these studies were compared with those of studies using drug therapy, it was apparent that the nondrug approach was as effective as drugs, and without side effects. These results clearly demonstrate that the primary therapy for migraine headaches should be relaxation. (See page 35 for a description of ways to create the relaxation response.)

My clinical experience indicates that food allergy or sensitivity plays a primary role in many migraine headaches. Many double-blind, placebo-controlled studies have demonstrated that the detection and removal of allergenic foods will eliminate or greatly reduce headache symptoms in the majority of patients, especially children. Food allergy or intolerance induces a migraine attack largely because platelets release compounds, such as serotonin and histamine, that lead to vascular instability. In addition, food additives and foods such as aged cheeses, beer, canned figs, chicken liver, chocolate, pickled fish, the pods of broad beans, red wine, and brewer's yeast contain compounds (e.g., histamine and tyramine) that can set off migraines in sensitive individuals by causing blood vessels to expand.[10, 11, 12, 13, 14]

Identify Food Allergies

Many nutritionally oriented physicians perform blood tests to diagnose food allergies. However, in most cases such tests are not really necessary. For patients who have to pay for such tests out of pocket, these tests can be expensive. My experience is that it is best to try a simple elimination diet for seven to 10 days first, to see if your symptoms improve. Start by eliminating the most common allergens:

- Milk and all dairy products
- Wheat (including wheat flour products—e.g., bread, pastries, pasta)
- Corn
- Citrus fruit (e.g., oranges, tangerines, lemons, and grapefruit)
- Peanuts and peanut butter
- Eggs
- Processed foods containing artificial food coloring

As part of an elimination diet, I also recommend using RevitalX—a high-potency multinutrient powdered drink mix from Natural Factors. This product was specifically developed by Michael Lyon, M.D., to be an excellent source of important nutrients to support the gastrointestinal lining and aid detoxification. In an allergy elimination diet, RevitalX is taken twice per day as the primary source of sustenance. RevitalX is mixed with water or juice (fresh vegetable juice is preferred), or it can be blended as a fruit smoothie. Fresh or steamed vegetables and small amounts of fruit can be eaten when you are hungry, and one simple meal is prepared in the evening: steamed vegetables, lean chicken breast, and brown rice (cooked beans, split peas, or lentils along with brown rice can be used as a vegetarian alternative). A lightly sautéed stir-fry can also be prepared for this meal.

If your symptoms disappear within seven to 10 days, you're on the right track. By slowly reintroducing the previously avoided foods back into the diet (for example, trying one "new" food every three days), and paying attention to which ones cause symptoms to return, you can identify the real culprit.

Will you be able to eat that food again? This depends on whether the allergy is cyclic or fixed. Cyclic allergies develop slowly and result from repeatedly eating a certain food. After the allergenic food has been avoided for a period of time (typically three to four months), it may be reintroduced. Usually the food won't cause symptoms again unless you eat it too frequently or in large amounts. Cyclic allergies account for roughly 80 to 90 percent of food allergies. Fixed allergies occur whenever a food is eaten, no matter how much time has passed. If you have a fixed allergy, you will remain allergic to the food for life.

Several natural products have shown impressive results in the treatment of migraine headaches:

- ▸ **Riboflavin.** One of the theories used to explain a migraine headache is that it is caused by reduced energy production within the mitochondria, units of cells of blood vessels in the head. Therefore, because vitamin B$_2$ (riboflavin) can potentially increase cellular energy production, it was thought that this vitamin might prevent migraine. In one double-blind study with riboflavin—400 milligrams (mg) daily—the proportion of patients who improved by at least 50 percent was 15 percent for a placebo and 59 percent for riboflavin.[15] There were no side effects attributed to the riboflavin therapy. It is notable that riboflavin is as nearly as effective as drugs for migraines, but is much safer and relatively cheap.

▸ **Magnesium.** An insufficiency of magnesium may also play a significant role in many headaches. Several researchers have demonstrated substantial links between low magnesium levels and both migraine and tension headaches. A magnesium deficiency is known to set the stage for the events that can cause a migraine attack or a tension headache.[16, 17] Low brain, tissue, and cellular concentrations of magnesium have been found in patients with migraines, indicating a need for supplementation, since a key function of magnesium is to maintain the tone of the blood vessels and prevent overexcitability of nerve cells. Magnesium supplementation can be quite effective in preventing migraine headaches.[18, 19] The recommended dosage is 150 to 250 mg three times daily. Magnesium bound to citrate, malate, or aspartate is better absorbed and better tolerated than inorganic forms such as magnesium sulfate, hydroxide, or oxide, which tend to have a laxative effect. An increased intake of high-magnesium foods such as nuts, tofu, and green leafy vegetables also makes a lot of sense.

▸ **Petadolex®.** This standardized extract from the butterbur plant (*Petasites hybridus*) has been shown in several double-blind studies to produce excellent results as a treatment for migraine headaches, without side effects.[20] In one study, 60 patients with headaches randomly received either 50 mg of Petadolex twice daily for 12 weeks, or a placebo.[21] Petadolex reduced the frequency of attacks by 46 percent after four weeks, 60 percent after eight weeks, and 50 percent after 12 weeks of treatment. (The results for the placebo group were:

24 percent, 17 percent, and 10 percent, respectively.) Petadolex is generally well tolerated, but diarrhea has been reported in some individuals. If this side effect occurs, discontinue use. Its safety during pregnancy and lactation has not been determined. The typical adult dosage ranges from 50 to 100 mg twice daily with meals.

THE INFECTION "EQUATION"

One of the most significant differences between a naturopathic physician and a conventional medical doctor becomes apparent when you take a look how each views and addresses an infection. Many doctors do not even consider the role of the immune system in the susceptibility to or treatment of an infection. They do not fully understand that the immune system, if functioning optimally, can adequately defend against virtually all infectious organisms except those that are particularly virulent.

Whether we develop an infection or not is a result of the strength of our defense mechanisms versus the virulence of the infective organism. An infection can be thought of, loosely, as like a mathematical equation, such as one plus two equals three. In an infection, what will determine the outcome is the interaction of the host's immune system with the infecting organism. A naturopathic doctor tends to use treatments designed to enhance the immune system, whereas most conventional doctors tend to use antibiotics designed to kill the infecting organism, even if antibiotic therapy has been shown to be of limited (if any) value.

Conventional medicine has been obsessed with killing the infective organism rather than promoting defense against infection. This obsession really began with Louis Pasteur, the nineteenth-century physician and researcher who played a major role in the development of germ theory. This theory holds that different diseases are caused by different infectious organisms. Much of Pasteur's life was dedicated to finding substances that would kill the infecting organisms. Pasteur and later figures who pioneered effective treatments for infectious diseases have given us a great deal for which we all should be thankful. However, there is more to the situation than the virility of the organism.

Another nineteenth-century French scientist, Claude Bernard, also made major contributions to medical understanding. But Bernard had a different view of health and disease. He believed that a person's internal environment was more important in determining disease than any infective organism or pathogen. In other words, he believed that the internal terrain or the host's susceptibility to infection was more important than the germ. Physicians, he believed, should focus more on making this internal terrain a very inhospitable place for disease.

Bernard's theory led to some rather interesting studies. In fact, a firm advocate of germ theory would consider some of these studies absolutely crazy. One of the most interesting was conducted by a Russian scientist, Élie Metchnikoff, the discover of the white blood cells. He and his research associates consumed cultures containing millions of cholera bacteria. Yet none of them developed cholera. The reason: their immune systems were not compromised. Metchnikoff believed, like Bernard, that the correct way to deal with infectious disease was to focus on enhancing the body's own defenses.

Late in their lives, Pasteur and Bernard engaged in scientific discussions on the virtues of the germ theory and Bernard's perspective on the internal terrain. Supposedly, on his deathbed, Pasteur said: "Bernard was right. The pathogen is nothing. The terrain is everything." Whether this is actually true or not, the point is that modern medicine has largely forgotten the importance of the "terrain."

THE WIDESPREAD ABUSE OF ANTIBIOTICS

Despite my belief that the focus should be on promoting the body's own defenses against infection, I want to make it very clear that antibiotics definitely have a place in modern medicine. In fact, I am extremely grateful that we have these wondrous agents available. When my daughter, Alexa, was 10 months old she developed a kidney infection from which she probably would not have recovered without antibiotics. There is little argument that when used appropriately antibiotics save lives. However, there is also little argument that antibiotics are grossly overused. The appropriate use of antibiotics makes good medical sense; what does not make sense is the reliance on antibiotics for such conditions as acne, recurrent bladder infections, chronic ear infections, chronic sinusitis, chronic bronchitis, and nonbacterial sore throats. Relying on antibiotics to treat these conditions does not make sense, because the antibiotics rarely provide real benefit.

Cold Remedies and Children

On October 19, 2007, a panel of the FDA voted 13 to 9 to recommend against the use of over-the-counter (OTC) cough and cold products for children under the age of six years. The panel has concluded that these popular medications offered no benefit and involved considerable risk. However, possibly yielding to the demands of drug manufacturers, the panel decided against making a similar recommendation for older children, even though earlier it had agreed there was no evidence that the products do any good for that age group, either.

The FDA is not bound by these conclusions, but it does usually follow the advice of its advisory panels. Officials of the FDA said they would review the complex recommendations and decide how to proceed. Because the products have been on the market so long, formal action could take years, the officials said. But the FDA plans to consult with the industry about possible voluntary action and whether to offer the public interim advice.

No one knows how many children have had adverse reactions to the medications, but the federal Centers for Disease Control and Prevention reported earlier in 2007 that at least 1,500 children younger than age two suffered complications in 2004 and 2005. A review prepared by the FDA for the October 2007 meeting described dozens of cases of convulsions, heart problems, trouble with breathing, neurological complications, and other reactions, including at least 123 deaths.

The hearing came a week after major manufacturers of the medications voluntarily withdrew 14 products designed for children younger than age two, including well-known brands such as Dimetapp Decongestant Plus Cough Infant Drops, Tylenol Concentrated Infants' Drops Plus Cold, and Robitussin Infant Cough DM Drops.

The widespread abuse of antibiotics is becoming increasingly alarming for many reasons, including a near-epidemic of chronic candidiasis and the development of superbugs that are resistant to currently available antibiotics. According to many experts as well as the World Health Organization (WHO), we are coming dangerously close to a post-antibiotic era when many infectious diseases will once again become almost impossible to treat.

Since there is evidence that resistance to antibiotics is less of a problem when antibiotics are used sparingly, prescribing fewer antibiotics may be the only significant way to address the problem. According to several authorities as well as WHO, antibiotics must be restricted and inappropriate uses must be halted if the growing trend toward bacterial resistance to antibiotics is to be stopped or reversed.

ASTHMA—A CONSEQUENCE OF ANTIBIOTICS

The rate of asthma in children has doubled in the last 10 to 15 years. Why? In a combined analysis of seven studies involving more than 12,000 youngsters, researchers at the University of British Columbia found that those who had taken prescribed antibiotics before their first birthday were more than twice as likely as untreated kids to develop asthma. Among children who had multiple courses of antibiotics, the risk was even higher—it rose 16 percent for every course of the drugs taken before age one.[22]

Again, there is no question that antibiotics have their place in medicine—they definitely save lives. But here is my point: the majority of these kids may have developed asthma from antibiotics given to them for conditions (e.g., bronchitis, ear infections, and colds) against which antibiotics have not been shown to be effective.

There are a couple of explanations for this association between antibiotics and asthma. One is that antibiotics contribute to a state of "excess hygiene" leading to a reduced exposure to microbes, which in turn creates an oversensitive immune system mounting an over-the-top allergic reaction to pollen and dust mites, ultimately leading to asthma.

My feeling is that the underlying mechanism explaining a possible link between antibiotics and asthma is the negative effect of antibiotics on the normal flora in the gastrointestinal and respiratory passages, as I explained in the last chapter. Recent clinical studies have shown that taking probiotics (active cultures of beneficial bacteria such as *Lactobacillus* and *Bifidobacteria* species) lowers the risk of allergic diseases like asthma and eczema. These results definitely indicate that antibiotics actively raise the risk by wiping out these beneficial bacteria.

ANTIBIOTICS AND ACUTE BRONCHITIS

Over the past 20 years there have been several randomized controlled trials designed to assess the benefit of antibiotics in treating acute bronchitis. Despite sufficient data (now more than a dozen double-blind studies) showing no clinical benefit for antibiotics in acute bronchitis, these drugs are prescribed by 70 percent of doctors who encounter a patient presenting with acute bronchitis. This practice is also in direct conflict with the practice guidelines of the American College of Chest Physicians—the medical specialty that deals with bronchitis and other respiratory disorders.[23] According to their most recent guidelines, "The widespread use of antibiotics for the treatment of acute bronchitis is not justified, and vigorous efforts to curtail their use should be encouraged." Nonetheless, most doctors regularly prescribe an antibiotic for acute bronchitis even though it provides no benefit and does have significant risks. The risks include overgrowth of *Candida albicans*, disruption of normal gut microflora, and the possibility of developing antibiotic-resistant strains of bacteria.

Why do physicians prescribe antibiotics for acute bronchitis despite the scientific facts? This is a very good question. Apparently, in addition to wanting to offer some help, doctors have several misconceptions. For example, there are no data to support the use of antibiotics when a patient's history is, "I've had a cough for a week, and now my phlegm has turned green." Likewise, there are no data to support the use of antibiotics because of a fever in acute bronchitis, or in the hope of preventing a progression to pneumonia. Another reason why doctors prescribe antibiotics for acute bronchitis is that many patients believe only an antibiotic can cure it. This belief is

perhaps best exemplified by the fact that 60 percent of eligible patients refused to enter one double-blind study because they felt that antibiotics were
absolutely necessary.[24] Given doctors' and patients' beliefs and expectations,
it is little wonder that antibiotics continue to be prescribed for a condition
whose course they will not alter and for which they are never warranted.

ANTIBIOTICS AND EAR INFECTIONS

The major reason for the use of antibiotics in childhood is the misguided
belief that they are necessary to treat ear infections. A number of well-
designed studies and detailed analyses have demonstrated that there were
no significant differences in the clinical course of acute ear infections between children treated with antibiotics and children given a placebo.[25, 26, 27]
Interestingly, in some studies, children who did *not* receive antibiotics had
fewer recurrences than children who received antibiotics. This result undoubtedly reflects the fact that antibiotics suppress the immune system and
disturb the normal flora of the upper respiratory tract. Despite the data
showing little, if any, benefit from antibiotics in treating ear infections, 98
percent of children with an ear infection in the United States are given an
antibiotic.

FOOD ALLERGIES AND EAR INFECTIONS

The primary risk factors for ear infections include:

▸ Food allergies

▸ Exposure to secondhand smoke

▸ Not being breast-fed

▸ Day care

▸ Pacifiers

All these factors can contribute to abnormal functioning of the eustachian tube, the underlying cause in virtually all cases of ear infections. The

eustachian tube connects the middle ear to the back of the inner throat. It functions to regulate gas pressure in the middle ear, protects the middle ear from nose and throat secretions and bacteria, and clears fluids from the middle ear. Swallowing causes active opening of the eustachian tube due to the action of the surrounding muscles. Infants and small children are particularly susceptible to problems of the eustachian tube because at their age it is smaller in diameter and more horizontal.

Obstruction of the eustachian tube leads first to fluid buildup and then, if the bacteria present are pathogenic and the immune system is impaired, to bacterial infection. Obstruction results from collapse of the tube (due to weak tissues holding the tube in place, or to an abnormal opening mechanism, or to both), blockage with mucus in response to allergy or irritation, swelling of the mucous membrane, or infection.

The role of allergy as a major cause of chronic ear infections has been demonstrated in numerous studies, but for some reason it remains controversial in conventional medical circles.[28, 29, 30, 31, 32] Studies have shown that 93 percent of children with ear infections have allergies: 16 percent to inhalants only, 14 percent to food only, and 70 percent to both. One way prolonged breast-feeding prevents ear infections may be by the avoidance of food allergies, particularly if the mother avoids sensitizing foods (i.e., those to which she is allergic) during pregnancy and lactation. In addition to breast-feeding, also of value is the exclusion or limited consumption of the foods to which children are most commonly allergic—wheat, egg, peanuts, corn, citrus, chocolate, and dairy products—particularly during the first nine months.

The allergic reaction causes blockage of the eustachian tube by two mechanisms: inflammatory swelling of the mucous membranes lining the tube, and inflammatory swelling of the nose, causing what is known as the Toynbee phenomenon (swallowing when both mouth and nose are closed, forcing air and secretions into the middle ear). In chronic ear infections, an allergy should always be considered as a possible cause, and any offending allergen should be identified and avoided. If that goal is achieved, the results are fabulous. For example, in one large study of children with chronic ear infections, after 12 months 92 percent improved when their allergies were identified and dealt with.[31] In another study, the success rate was 78 percent.[32] In contrast, the typical response with conventional medical treatment—antibiotics or surgical methods, including ear tubes and the removal of the tonsils and adenoids—is only about 50 percent.

WHAT'S A PARENT TO DO?

The point that I want to make here is that the best medicine is always prevention. Helping your child build a strong immune system is the primary goal. Breast-feeding for at least the first four months of life, avoiding food allergies and airborne irritants (such as cigarette smoke), and providing optimum nutrition are all very important in helping children develop greater resistance to infections. When illness does present itself, visiting a naturopathic physician for natural support should be the first step (please go to www.naturopathic.org to find an N.D. in your area).

In the treatment of acute ear infections, an eardrop preparation containing various herbal medicines was shown to be very effective in reducing pain and calming a crying child.[33] In a double-blind trial with 171 children ages 5 to 18, eardrops containing a combination of extracts of marigold flowers (*Calendula officinalis*), St.-John's-wort (*Hypericum perforatum*), and mullein flowers (*Verbascum thapsus*) in olive oil with the essential oil of garlic (*Allium sativum*) were given at a dose of five drops in the affected ear three times daily to the experimental group. This treatment was compared with the same dosage of an anesthetic eardrops containing amethocaine and phenazone. Other children were given either no antibiotic or amoxicillin. All the groups had a statistically significant improvement in ear pain over the course of three days, but the group getting the herbal eardrops without an antibiotic had the best response: a 95.9 percent reduction in their pain score. If the herbal eardrops were given with amoxicillin there was a 90.9 percent diminution of pain. The children given the anesthetic drops alone and with antibiotics had reductions of 84.7 percent and 77.8 percent, respectively. These data indicate that the topical treatment with herbal eardrops was the most effective.

ANOTHER EXAMPLE OF MORE
HARM THAN GOOD

There are many effective alternatives to conventional drugs, but perhaps the best-known is the dietary supplement glucosamine sulfate in the treatment of osteoarthritis. Often, what is different about using such natural alternatives is that they truly promote the healing process rather than suppress symptoms. There is probably no better example than comparing the natural approach and the drug approach to osteoarthritis—the most common form of arthritis.

Osteoarthritis is characterized by a breakdown of cartilage. Cartilage has an important role in joint function. Its gel-like consistency provides protection to the ends of joints by acting as a shock absorber. Degeneration of the cartilage is the defining feature of osteoarthritis. This degeneration causes inflammation, pain, deformity, and limitation of motion in the joint.

Several studies have attempted to determine the natural course of osteoarthritis.[34, 35] In other words, researchers have sought to determine what happens when people with osteoarthritis are given no treatment. One group of researchers studied the natural course of osteoarthritis of the hip over a 10-year period.[35] At the beginning of the study, all subjects had X-rays suggestive of advanced osteoarthritis, yet the researchers reported marked clinical improvement over time. X-rays confirmed these improvements, including complete recovery in 14 of 31 subjects. These results, as well as others, raise the serious concern that medical intervention (i.e., drugs) may actually promote the progression of this disease.

KNEE SURGERY FOR OSTEOARTHRITIS
IS NO BETTER THAN A PLACEBO

In a landmark study conducted by Baylor College of Medicine, a popular surgical treatment for osteoarthritis was shown to provide no real benefit.[36] The procedure involves the use of an arthroscope, a pencil-thin viewing tube. With the arthroscope, worn, torn, or loose cartilage is cut away and removed (debridement); or the bad cartilage is simply washed away (lavaged). In the study, 180 patients with knee pain were randomized into three groups. One group received debridement; the second group underwent arthroscopic lavage; and the third group underwent simulated arthroscopic surgery—small incisions were made, but no instruments were inserted and no cartilage was removed.

During two years of follow-up, patients in all three groups reported moderate improvements in pain and ability to function. However, neither of the intervention groups reported less pain or better function than the placebo group. In fact, the placebo patients reported better outcomes than the debridement patients at certain points during follow-up. Throughout the two years, the patients were unaware of whether they had received real or placebo surgery.

In the United States, it is estimated that more than 650,000 arthroscopic debridement or lavage procedures are performed each year. At a cost of about $5,000 each, they represent roughly $3.25 billion. That is a lot of money, which could be put to better use than in a therapy that provides no real benefit to the patient.

DRUGS USED IN OSTEOARTHRITIS CAN PROMOTE JOINT DESTRUCTION

The primary drugs used in the treatment of osteoarthritis are the nonsteroidal anti-inflammatory drugs (NSAIDs). They include aspirin, ibuprofen, Aleve, Feldene, Voltarin, and the newer COX-2 inhibitor drugs such as Celebrex and Vioxx. These drugs are used extensively in the United States in the treatment of osteoarthritis, but research is indicating that they may be producing only short-term benefit and actually accelerating joint destruction and causing more problems down the road. These drugs are also associated with side effects, including gastrointestinal upset, headaches, and dizziness, and are therefore recommended for only short periods of time. In Chapter 1, I emphasized that although Celebrex and Vioxx came into prominence precisely to avoid the ulcers caused by anti-inflammatory drugs like aspirin and ibuprofen, after one year of use there was actually no differ-

Vioxx Costs Merck Billions

When Merck Pharmaceuticals announced on September 20, 2004, that it was voluntarily withdrawing its arthritis medication Vioxx (which had been worth $2.5 billion a year) from the market because of the risk of heart attacks, it highlighted once again the failure of the FDA to adequately protect Americans from the greed and manipulation of the drug companies. It was not the loss of lives per se that was responsible for Merck's withdrawing the drug and losing billions of dollars in revenues. Rather, it was probably a fear of the financial damages that a major class action law suit would inflict on Merck.

Merck's executives were no doubt keenly aware of results of class action lawsuits involving the drug Baycol (cerivastatin), manufactured by the German drug company Bayer. This statin was shown to produce an often fatal destruction of muscle tissue (rhabdomyolysis) more than 20 times as frequently as other statin drugs. From the time Bayer became aware of the problem, one year elapsed before Baycol was removed from the market in August 2001; during that year there were 1,899 cases of rhabdomyolysis and at least 100 deaths. Bayer has paid $1.133 billion to settle 2,995 cases worldwide, and nearly 10,000 cases are still pending.

Can you imagine the deep concern the makers of Vioxx had when reports began to surface that COX-2 inhibitor drugs such as Vioxx and Celebrex might be linked to as many as 50,000 deaths in the United States alone? In the debacle over Baycol, Bayer paid on average $381,224 to each claimant. If family members of the victims of Vioxx received similar compensation, it would clearly bankrupt Merck, especially in light of the fact that Merck apparently was aware of the potential link between Vioxx and heart attacks. The removal of Vioxx from the market was mainly an attempt by Merck to reduce its liability. Even so, by March 2006, more than 10,000 cases and 190 class actions were filed against Merck, involving adverse cardiovascular events associated with Vioxx and the inadequacy of Merck's warnings. In the first case to go all the way to trial, on August 19, 2005, a jury in Texas voted 10 to two to hold Merck liable for the death of Robert Ernst at age 59. The jury awarded his wife, Carol Ernst, $253.4 million in damages. But she will have a tough time getting that money, as Merck will appeal and fight this case and any other case it might lose. Merck has set aside nearly $1 billion to pay for legal expenses related to Vioxx.

ence between Celebrex and the older drugs ibuprofen and Voltaren with re-gard to the formation of ulcers. In light of the subsequent disclosures about Celebrex and Vioxx, and because it is estimated that more than 60,000 peo-ple may have died from side effects of these drugs, it seems that the drugs should never have been approved for use.

One side effect of these NSAIDs that the drug companies won't tell you about and your doctor doesn't know about is that they can actually promote joint destruction and inhibit cartilage repair by inhibiting the formation of key compounds in cartilage, the glycosaminoglycans (GAGs).[37] These com-pounds are responsible for maintaining the proper water content in the cartilage matrix, thereby helping cartilage remain gel-like and continue to absorb shock. Clinical studies have shown that NSAIDs are associated with acceleration of osteoarthritis and increased joint destruction.[38, 39, 40, 41] Sim-ply stated, aspirin and other NSAIDs appear to suppress the symptoms but accelerate the progression of osteoarthritis. They are designed to fight dis-ease rather than promote health.

GLUCOSAMINE SULFATE IN THE TREATMENT OF OSTEOARTHRITIS

Glucosamine is a simple molecule that can be manufactured in the body. In joints, the main function of glucosamine is to stimulate the manufacture of glycosaminoglycans (GAGs), structural components of cartilage. Evidently, as some people age they lose the ability to manufacture sufficient levels of glucosamine. The result is that cartilage loses its capacity to act as a shock absorber. The inability to manufacture glucosamine has been suggested as the major factor leading to osteoarthritis—the most common form of ar-thritis, characterized by joint degeneration and loss of cartilage.

The most thoroughly researched form of glucosamine is glucosamine sulfate. This form has been the subject of more than 300 scientific investiga-tions and at least 20 double-blind studies. Glucosamine sulfate has been used by millions of people worldwide, has no known toxicity in humans, and is registered as drug in the treatment of osteoarthritis in some 70 coun-tries.[42, 43, 44]

The medicinal use of glucosamine sulfate in the treatment of osteoarthritis is consistent with the philosophy and practice of naturopathic medicine because of its action in facilitating the body's natural healing process.
The clinical benefits of glucosamine sulfate in the treatment of osteoarthritis are impressive. In comparative studies it has been shown to provide
greater benefit than NSAIDs such as ibuprofen and piroxicam (Feldene).
Although side effects are common (even expected) with these drugs, glucosamine sulfate does not cause side effects. One popular misconception
that I have heard from both doctors and consumers is that glucosamine sulfate raises blood sugar levels. It is true that according to test-tube studies
glucosamine can interfere with glucose metabolism. But, the concentrations used in these test-tube studies were 100 to 200 times higher than tissue levels that can be reached with oral supplementation. When researchers
went back and reviewed clinical trials involving more than 3,000 subjects,
they found that fasting blood sugar levels actually decreased slightly with
use of glucosamine sulfate.[44]

In studies comparing glucosamine sulfate with ibuprofen, piroxicam
(Feldene), or acetaminophen, results have shown glucosamine sulfate was
more effective in relieving pain (though it does not have any direct analgesic
effect) and was without significant side effects. In fact, subjects on glucosamine sulfate had fewer side effects than subjects in the placebo, and
there were no dropouts in the glucosamine sulfate group. In contrast, many
of the subjects taking NSAIDs had side effects and dropped out because
these side effects are so severe.

In summary, whereas NSAIDs and acetaminophen offer only symptomatic relief in osteoarthritis and may actually promote the disease process,
glucosamine sulfate appears to address one of the underlying factors that
can cause osteoarthritis—reduced manufacture of the components of cartilage. Clinical studies have now confirmed that glucosamine sulfate can actually thicken cartilage, thereby restoring its shock-absorbing qualities. By
getting at the root of the problem, glucosamine sulfate not only improves
the symptoms, including pain, but also helps the body repair damaged joints.
The treatment of osteoarthritis is just one instance in which a more natural
approach produces better results and does so without side effects.

Case History: The Plumber's Helper

Jack, a 56-year-old plumber, could barely walk into my office because his knee hurt so much. He told me that he had dragged himself in because he had read an article I had written on the value of glucosamine sulfate over NSAIDs in the treatment of osteoarthritis.

Jack had learned firsthand how destructive these drugs can be. About 10 years before, he started developing osteoarthritis in his left knee. His medical doctor first offered a prescription for ibuprofen (Motrin). When that didn't work, the doctor prescribed more potent NSAIDs, including Voltaren and Feldene. In the 10 years he had taken these drugs, Jack's arthritis got worse. Adding insult to injury, a severe ulcer developed in his stomach.

Two weeks before coming to me, Jack had been hospitalized because his ulcer was bleeding. Because his stomach was so bad, he had to stop taking Feldene. When he stopped, his knee hurt worse than ever. The acetaminophen (Tylenol) his doctor now prescribed was not working. Jack grew desperate and began looking into other options. That's when he read my article about natural alternatives for dealing with osteoarthritis, but he was such a skeptic that he wanted to hear it directly from the horse's mouth. He simply could not imagine that treating osteoarthritis could be as simple as I professed. I told him that it did not matter if he believed that glucosamine sulfate would work or not—I knew it would. Jack agreed to try.

When he returned six weeks later, he was ecstatic. He was doing deep knee bends and hopping up and down on his left leg to show me how good he felt. He said it was a miracle. He felt so good that the day before he had gone to his medical doctor's office to show off his progress with glucosamine sulfate. His doctor said it was nothing more than a placebo response. Jack had replied, "Doc, if it was just a placebo, then why didn't you prescribe it to me ten years ago instead of giving me all of those damn drugs?" I think Jack had a good point.

Jack came to see me in 1995, when glucosamine sulfate was just hitting the market. Most doctors at the time were not familiar with the science behind glucosamine sulfate. So, I sent Jack's doctor a packet of information on glucosamine sulfate, including reports on several of the double-blind, placebo-controlled trials. A week later I received a very nice letter from the doctor. He thanked me and stated that he was unaware of all the double-blind studies supporting the efficacy of glucosamine sulfate. He was also surprised to learn that glucosamine sulfate is an approved medicine in more than 70 countries and has been used successfully by millions of people worldwide. My experience is that most conventional medical doctors appreciate learning about safe and effective tools that can help their patients.

FINAL COMMENTS

So, is relieving symptoms a path to bad medicine? My answer to this question is yes, but with some clarification. Relief of symptoms should be a major therapeutic goal, but it should not come at the price of doing more harm than good. Whether relief of symptoms is good or bad is determined by whether the treatment simply suppresses the symptoms or eliminates the underlying factors that are producing them. Symptoms are often whistle-blowers, alerting us to deeper issues. The whistle-blower is silenced, but this does not necessarily mean that the deeper issue has been taken care of. Think of a fire alarm: if you simply turn it off, the fire may burn out of control. Don't underestimate the wisdom of your body or its ability to sense when something is not right. Symptoms often provide us with valuable information so that we can make changes that will lead to better health.

6

CREATING A MARKET VERSUS PROVIDING A CURE

"Once a upon a time, drug companies promoted drugs to treat disease. Now it is often just the opposite. They promote diseases to fit their drugs."

—Marcia Angell, M.D., former editor in chief of the *New England Journal of Medicine* and author of *The Truth about Drug Companies*

LET'S FACE IT: DRUG companies are driven by the goal of generating dollars, and they are committed to doing whatever needs to be done to get their drugs to market. And once a drug is on the market, they will do just about anything necessary to sell it to physicians and the public through manipulation, hiring the right experts, and spending enormous amounts of money on advertising campaigns and on inducements to doctors to prescribe it. In their world, money is not everything; it is the only thing.

The ideal for a drug company would be to develop a drug that could address a condition everyone has and then convince doctors and the public that this drug approach is the only way to deal with the condition. Much has been written about the pharmaceutical industry's goal of turning us all into patients by using its influence to narrows the limits of what is considered "normal." Perhaps the best examples of this approach were convincing doctors that the natural process of menopause was in fact a "disease" requiring medical treatment in the form of hormone replacement therapy (HRT); convincing doctors that osteoporosis must be treated with drugs so as to prevent hip fractures; and convincing them that lowering cholesterol levels with statin drugs is an effective way to increase life expectancy by preventing heart disease in the general public (this last topic is discussed in Chapter 7).

WOMEN AS GUINEA PIGS

In 1966, Robert A. Wilson, M.D., introduced, in his book *Feminine Forever*, the theory that menopause is an estrogen deficiency disease caused by the normal decline of estrogen with aging, and that it needs to be treated with estrogen to compensate for this decline. According to Wilson, without estrogen replacement therapy, women are destined to become sexless "caricatures of their former selves . . . the equivalent of a eunuch."

Although menopause is a natural process—the term simply denotes the cessation of menstruation in women—Wilson's theory of menopause as a disease became the dominant medical view until about 2002. In that year, the National Institutes of Health (NIH) halted a major clinical trial designed to help settle the debate over whether HRT benefits postmenopausal women. This study, the Women's Health Initiative (WHI), concluded that the risks of taking combined estrogen and progestin outweighed the benefits; the therapy increased the risk of stroke, coronary heart disease, and breast cancer. The findings that led researchers to pull the plug early on WHI included links between HRT and:

- a 26 percent increase in invasive breast cancer

- a 41 percent increase in strokes

- a 29 percent increase in heart attacks

- a doubling of the rate of blood clots in legs and lungs

- a twofold to threefold increase in gallstones and liver disease[1]

Once the awareness of the dangers of HRT increased, many doctors and the public became aware of the other studies reporting similar alarming statistics. For example, HRT not only stimulates the growth of invasive breast cancers but also makes it harder to spot the potentially deadly tumors on mammograms; HRT doubled the risk of developing Alzheimer's disease; and HRT increased the risk of life-threatening blood clots.

The WHI was viewed as a major revelation of the risks and inefficacy of HRT, but in reality this study and others to follow only confirmed was what already known from previous studies about the dangers of these synthetic versions of natural hormones.[2, 3, 4, 5, 6] A year or so before WHI was halted, I spoke to at least 400 M.D.s about natural approaches to menopause, at a medical conference. Part of my presentation included sharing the facts on HRT. I could see from the reaction of my audience that the information was not being well received, and during the question-and-answer period it was quite apparent that I had hit a very sensitive nerve. I simply shared with these doctors that when all the studies are examined collectively, it could be concluded that HRT was associated with as much as a 30 percent increase in the risk of breast cancer and that there was little (if any) protective effect against heart disease. Interestingly, at that time—2001— most of the studies linking HRT to breast cancer were conducted in Europe. In comparison, up to 2001 only a few studies in the United States showed that HRT increased the risk of breast cancer. The difference in the link between HRT and breast cancer in the early studies raised some interesting questions for me. Are American researchers biased? Some studies of American women showed no increased risk of breast cancer: was this outcome due to the fact that American women are already at a high risk for breast cancer? Also, why are American researchers and doctors so defensive about the link to breast cancer found in the European studies?

I have lectured to medical doctors for more than 20 years. In general, my presentations have been very well received. But the response that I elicited with this lecture was unlike any other. The doctors bristled when I presented evidence that HRT was not all it was cracked up to be. Why this reaction? I realized that most of these doctors, like most other doctors in the United States, had been enthusiastically recommending HRT to their female patients for many, many years. No well-intentioned researchers or physicians want to admit that a drug that they have been strongly supporting could be irrefutably linked to a dreaded disease such as breast cancer and to an increased risk of death from cardiovascular disease.

The doctors had been influenced by marketing and "conventional wisdom" rather than science. There was absolutely no solid clinical evidence that HRT had a protective effect against cardiovascular disease, but during my question-and-answer session that supposed protection was said to offset the link to breast cancer. Yes, the doctors seemed to agree that HRT does increase the risk of breast cancer, but this risk is offset by a reduction in heart attack and strokes, so life expectancy actually increases. The discussion became very heated when I kept pointing out that the cardioprotective effect of these synthetic hormones was a myth propagated by the drug companies, and that the available clinical studies actually showed an increase in cardiovascular disease with HRT. In the end, we all agreed that the answer to the entire issue would be put to rest by WHI. Of course, when WHI was halted and the results were published, I was quick to point it out, in an e-mail to the sponsors of the conference, that HRT actually increased strokes by 41 percent and heart attacks by 29 percent. In sum, HRT never had any real benefit other than relief of menopausal symptoms—and such relief is easily attained, without risk, through appropriate dietary, lifestyle, and supplemental strategies.

WHY IS HRT STILL BEING PRESCRIBED?

As damning as the results are, from WHI as well as from other studies on the long-term effects of HRT, it is a sad fact that approximately 30 million prescriptions for HRT were still being filled each year after 2002. That represents only about a 50 percent reduction compared with the year 2001 (pre-WHI). Why would doctors continue to prescribe HRT? Unfortunately, they are not aware of effective natural strategies to deal with menopausal symptoms or reduce the risk of osteoporosis.

As I tried to illustrate in Chapter 5, the suppression of symptoms is often a path to bad medicine. There is no question that HRT is effective at

Decrease in Breast Cancer Rates
Related to Reduction in Use of HRT

The immediate effect of WHI was a sudden drop in the number of women using HRT. Not surprisingly, there was a parallel sharp decline in the rate of new breast cancer cases.[7] Keep in mind that prior to 2002, breast cancer rates in the United States had been climbing steadily.

Prescriptions for the two most commonly prescribed forms of HRT in the United States—Premarin and Prempro—dropped from 61 million written in 2001 to 21 million in 2004. This drop was accompanied by a reduction of 8.4 percent in the annual rate of breast cancer in the United States. The decrease occurred only among women over the age of 50 and was more evident with cancers that were estrogen receptor (ER)–positive. These cancers need estrogen in order to grow and multiply. The speed at which breast cancer rates declined after the announcements regarding WHI may indicate that extremely small ER-positive breast cancers may have stopped progressing, or even regressed, after HRT was stopped. Clearly, this dramatic drop in the breast cancer rate further strengthens the link between breast cancer and use of HRT.

relieving the symptoms of menopause, but it is the opinion of many health experts (including me) that for most women long-term HRT is rarely justified: the risks outweigh the benefits. The only possible exception are women who are at high risk of developing osteoporosis. In the WHI study women receiving HRT had a 34 percent lower risk of hip fractures—one of the major consequences of osteoporosis. But there are also natural approaches to osteoporosis that can dramatically reduce the risk of this bone disease.

My recommendations for HRT have been consistent for more than two decades. It should consist only of natural "bioidentical" estrogen and progesterone, and it should be used only for menopausal women showing signs of, or having a significant risk of, osteoporosis, or for women who have severe menopausal symptoms that are not responsive to the natural, nonhormonal approach described below. To determine your risk of osteoporosis, and for more information on natural approaches, see Appendix B.

Major Risk Factors for Osteoporosis in Women

Being postmenopausal

Being white or Asian

Premature menopause

Positive family history

Short stature and small bones

Leanness

Low calcium intake

Inactivity

Being nulliparous (i.e., never having borne a child)

Gastric or small-bowel resection

Long-term glucocorticosteroid therapy

Long-term use of anticonvulsants

Hyperparathyroidism

Hyperthyroidism

Smoking

Heavy alcohol use

DANGEROUS FORMS OF HORMONES

Most women on HRT have no idea that they are taking unnatural forms of estrogen and progesterone. Premarin, for example, consists of forms of estrogen isolated from mare's urine (the name comes from pregnant mares' urine) and, all told, more than 200 substances mostly foreign to a human. Animal rights activists have longed claimed that the methods used to produce Premarin cause suffering to the mares. (Premarin is produced and collected at special pregnant mare urine—PMU—farms, and somewhat barbaric methods are involved.) The major health problem for women taking Premarin and other common forms of conjugated estrogens is that they are metabolized in the body to 17-beta-estradiol—the major carcinogenic form of estrogen. Synthetic versions of progesterone, such as megesterol, norethindrone, and norgestrel, used in HRT are perhaps even more problematic than conjugated estrogens.

If HRT is to be prescribed, it should be what is now referred to as "bioidentical" hormone replacement therapy (BHRT). The hormone components of BHRT are structurally identical to the natural forms of estrogen and progesterone produced in the human body. Because bioidentical hormones are natural, they are not patentable—hence, no big drug companies are promoting BHRT. There are some small studies indicating that BHRT is safer than, and as effective as, HRT in relieving menopausal symptoms; but without the promise of a financial windfall it is highly unlikely that the large trials necessary to conclusively show the advantages of bioidentical hormones will ever be conducted. Hence, although theoretically BHRT should be safer and more effective than HRT in long-term studies, the rational approach is to use BHRT only if it is necessary.

NATURAL HORMONE REPLACEMENT THERAPY

Most naturopathic physicians prefer to use a type of estrogen formulation known as triple estrogen, or Tri-Est, along with natural progesterone. Tri-Est provides a combination of the three major natural forms of estrogen: estriol, estrone, and estradiol in a ratio of 80:10:10. Estradiol is the principal estrogen found in a woman's body during the reproductive years, but it is also the form linked to breast cancer. The estrogen making up 80 percent of Tri-Est is estriol, a form associated with some protection against breast cancer. The concept behind Tri-Est is to provide estrogens similar to those your body produces but to give lower dosages of the stronger estrogens (estrone and estradiol) and higher levels of estriol. In this way, menopausal symptoms are relieved, and you fight osteoporosis and possibly offset the risk of breast cancer. The typical dosage of Tri-Est is 1.25 milligrams (mg) twice a day to treat mild to moderate symptoms; on 2.5 mg twice a day for moderate to severe symptoms.

Tri-Est and other natural combinations of estrogens are available by prescription through compounding pharmacies (pharmacies that compound or make the drugs on the premises). To find a compounding pharmacy in your area, and for more information, contact the International Academy of Compounding Pharmacists, www.iacprx.org, 1-800-927-4227.

If your doctor is averse to prescribing natural hormones from a compounding pharmacy, there are a number of bioidentical forms of estradiol available, including Estrace, Estrogel, Estraderm, Vivelle, Climara, Alora, Esclim, Orthoest, Ogen cream, Vagifem cream, and Estring. My recommendation if you are using one of these products, is to choose the topical cream or patch version. Applying estradiol to the skin is preferable to taking it orally, for several reasons, but primarily because a skin application appears to be considerably safer. This method more accurately approximates a woman's own natural estrogen secretions by delivering estradiol into the bloodstream in a slow, sustained manner and avoiding rapid breakdown by the liver.

The preferred progesterone is micronized natural progesterone. "Micronized" means that the hormone has been reduced to very small particles, which are easier to absorb. Micronized progesterone is available in tablets (e.g., Prometrium) as well as in creams. Avoid synthetic progestins such as megestrol, norethindrone, and norgestrel, as well as medroxyprogesterone acetate (e.g., Provera). Again, topical preparations are generally preferred.

NONHORMONAL APPROACHES TO MENOPAUSAL SYMPTOMS

The most common complaints during menopause are hot flashes, headaches, vaginal atrophy, frequent urinary tract infections, cold hands and feet, forgetfulness, and an inability to concentrate. Of these symptoms, hot flashes deserve the most attention. A hot flash is typically experienced as a feeling of intense heat with sweating and rapid heartbeat, and may last from two to 30 minutes. In the United States, 65 to 80 percent of menopausal women experience hot flashes to some degree. In contrast, studies of meno-pausal women in many traditional cultures throughout the world, and in Japan, have found that most of these women will pass through menopause without hot flashes. In addition, osteoporosis is extremely rare, despite the fact that the average woman in many traditional societies lives longer after menopause than women in the United States. Here are some effective natu-ral approaches for dealing with hot flashes.

► Exercise: Regular physical exercise definitely reduces the frequency and severity of hot flashes. In one study, women who spent an average of 3.5 hours per week exercising had no hot flashes whatsoever, whereas women who exercised less were more likely to have hot flashes.[8]

► Diet: The most important dietary recommendation may be to increase the consumption of plant foods, especially those high in phytoestrogens, while reducing the consumption of animal foods. Phytoestrogens are plant-derived substances that are able to weakly bind to the estrogen receptors in mammals and have a very weak, estrogen-like effect in some tissues and a weak antiestrogen effect in other tissues. Soybeans and flaxseeds have a high content of phytoestrogens. Many other foods, such as other legumes, apples, carrots, fennel, celery, and parsley, contain smaller amounts of phytoestrogens. A high dietary intake of phytoestrogens is thought to explain why hot flashes and other menopausal symptoms appear to occur less frequently in cultures consuming a predominantly plant-based diet. In addition, such a diet is promising for disease prevention; some research shows a lower incidence of breast, colon, and prostate cancer in those consuming high-phytoestrogen diets.[9, 10]

► Soy: Some clinical studies have shown eating soy foods (the equivalent of ⅔ cup of soybeans daily) to be effective in relieving hot flashes and vaginal atrophy.[11, 12] Not all studies show a consistent benefit, but when an increased soy intake helps reduce hot flashes or night sweats, it is generally in the range of a 30 percent to 55 percent reduction in these symptoms. This means that soy can help, but it is not likely to eliminate hot flashes. Currently, many soy products can be found in most grocery stores, and some unusual ones can be found in natural foods stores. They include dried soybeans, soy oil, soy milk, soy flour, roasted soy nuts, tofu, tofu pâté, tempeh, miso, soy sauce, natto, edamame, soy ice cream, soy cheese, soy candy bars, soy burgers and hot dogs, and soy marshmallows. The active components of soy are thought to be phytoestrogens known as isoflavones, but there is evidence that eating soy foods is more effective than taking soy isoflavone supplements.[12] Nonetheless, supplements containing soy isoflavones can also be used to deal with menopausal symptoms as well as possibly promote bone and cardiovascular health.[13, 14] The dosage should be in the same range as the dietary level of isoflavones in the traditional Asian diet, i.e., 45 to 90 mg per day of isoflavones. Again, my experience is that soy can help, but it is not strong enough on its own to eliminate hot flashes. For the greatest benefit, I would recommend focusing on dietary sources rather than taking a supplement.

▶ Flaxseeds: Flaxseeds contain lignans, a different class of phyto-estrogens. These are fiber compounds that can bind to estrogen receptors. Possibly, they help reduce menopausal symptoms and at the same time interfere with the carcinogenic effects of estrogen on breast tissue. Clinical studies in both premenopausal and postmenopausal women show that flaxseed can improve the body's ability to metabolize estrogen in a manner associated with a reduced risk of breast cancer.[15, 16] The best and by far the easiest way to gain the benefits of flaxseed is to use FortiFlax from Barlean's Organic Oils. This product is available at most health food stores; it contains ground flaxseeds in a special nitrogen-flushed container for maximum freshness. Grinding makes flaxseed lignans more bioavailable. Take 1 or 2 tablespoons daily. It can be easily added to foods like salads, smoothies, spreads, and yogurt.

Also, you can choose one or more of the following:

▸ Black cohosh (*Cimicifuga racemosa*). Black cohosh extract is the most well-researched and most popular herbal treatment for menopausal symptoms. Many, but not all, studies show very positive results.[17, 18, 19, 20] For example, in one study, when 80 patients were given either black cohosh extract (two tablets twice daily, providing 4 mg of 27-deoxyacteine daily) conjugated estrogens (0.625 mg daily), or a placebo for 12 weeks, the black cohosh extract produced the best results.[17] The number of hot flashes experienced each day dropped from an average of five to less than one in the group taking black cohosh. In comparison, flashes dropped from 5 to 3.5 in the group taking estrogen. Even more impressive was the effect of black cohosh on building up the vaginal lining. The dosage of black cohosh extract used in the majority of clinical studies has been enough to provide 2 mg of 27-deoxyacteine twice daily. I prefer to recommend herbal combination products for menopause that provide additional components such as dong quai (*Angelica sinensis*) and chaste berry (*Vitex agnus-castus*). However, the dosage of these products is still based on delivering the effective dosage of 2 mg of 27-deoxyacteine twice daily from black cohosh.

▸ Red clover (*Trifolium pratense*) extract. Red clover is very rich in phytoestrogens similar in action to soy isoflavones. Promensil is a patented red clover extract that has shown beneficial effects in some double-blind studies in women with menopausal symptoms at a dosage of 40 to 80 mg daily.[21, 22]

▸ Gamma-oryzanol (ferulic acid). This compound is found in grains and isolated from rice bran oil. Gamma-oryzanol was first shown to be effective for menopausal symptoms, including hot flashes, in the early 1960s. Subsequent studies have further documented its safety and effectiveness. In one study, 85 percent of the subjects who took 300 mg daily reported improvement in menopausal symptoms.[23]

Tapering Off HRT

If you elect to discontinue HRT in favor of the natural approach, the best (i.e., the most comfortable) method is to follow the dietary and supplementation strategies above for two weeks and then reduce the dosage of HRT by half. Continue at this half dosage for one month, then cut the dosage in half again by taking it every other day for another month before discontinuing it entirely.

WHAT ABOUT OSTEOPOROSIS DRUGS?

Osteoporosis means "porous bone." It involves both the mineral (inorganic) components of bone and the nonmineral components (organic matrix, composed primarily of protein). Bone is dynamic living tissue that is continually being broken down and rebuilt, even in adults. Osteoporosis occurs when more bone is breaking down than is being formed.

Osteoporosis currently affects between 13 percent and 30 percent of all postmenopausal women in the United States, depending on what criteria you use to define it. The most serious consequence of osteoporosis is fractures. It is estimated that osteoporosis causes approximately 1.5 million fractures every year. Of these, 250,000 are fractures of the hip. Despite the considerable advances in medical care, as many as 20 percent of women with hip fractures die within a year of the fracture, and 25 percent require long-term nursing care. Approximately half the women who suffer from a hip fracture are unable to walk without assistance. Obviously, one important goal in dealing with osteoporosis is to avoid hip fractures.

Though osteoporosis is largely a disease of diet and lifestyle, the drug industries have developed drugs for it. One class of drugs, the bisphosphonates, work by destroying a type of bone cell (osteoclast) responsible for remodeling bone, leading to an overall decrease in the breakdown of bone. Examples of bisphosphonates include Fosamax, Aredia, Boniva, Actonel, and Zometa.

In addition to the bisphophonates, there is a newer class of osteoporosis drugs, selective estrogen modulators (SERMs). The first of these drugs to be marketed was Evista (raloxifene). The SERMs work like a weak estrogen to stop bone loss. But since (unlike estrogen) they do not stimulate the breast or uterus, they are not associated with an increased risk of cancer. Interestingly, soy isoflavones act in a similar manner to reduce bone loss, but without side effects.

MARKETING FEAR

The evolution of the bisphosphonate empire began with Merck's Fosamax in 1995. As with many other blockbuster drugs, the growth in sales of Fosamax is a case study in effective manipulation by the drug companies. Apparently, the first step was a new definition of osteoporosis by the World Health Organization (WHO). No doubt led by experts who were sponsored by drug companies, WHO defined "normal" bone density as that of a 30-year old woman. Since there is a natural decline in bone density associated with aging, this new criterion immediately defined 30 percent of postmenopausal women as having osteoporosis.

Next, even before Fosamax reached the market, Merck was priming the pump by subsidizing the distribution of machines to test bone density. The strategy was simple. With the new guidelines in place and more accessible testing methods available, more prescriptions for Fosamax would be written. Merck worked hard to increase awareness (i.e., fear) of osteoporosis and impel women to get free bone density tests offered by local hospitals, clinics, and mobile facilities. The strategy worked perfectly. By 2003, Americans spent $1.7 billion annually on Fosamax.

Are such drugs effective? And what about their safety? Before answering these questions, I think it is important to answer the question, "Does testing bone mineral density help to prevent hip fractures?" The answer is quite interesting because once again it is contrary to conventional wisdom. According to a careful review of the literature and the results of a very large study, there is no correlation between testing alone and the prediction or prevention of fractures.[23] It seems that the test is not sensitive enough, because bone density is not the only risk factor that contributes to fractures.

In fact, osteoporosis accounts for only about 15 to 30 percent of all hip fractures in postmenopausal women. About one-third of all women who fracture a hip have normal bone density, and the rest are somewhere in between. Other important risk factors for hip fracture are a small frame, a low body mass index (BMI), long-term glucocorticoid therapy, cigarette smoking, excess alcohol intake, diabetes, family history, and conditions that increase the risk of falling, such as poor balance and muscular weakness.[24] For many patients, efforts to prevent falls by improving diet, lifestyle, balance, and muscular strength maybe more important in preventing fractures than increasing bone strength is.[25]

DETERMINING BONE MINERAL DENSITY

Bone mineral density (BMD) testing alone may not be a good predictor of fractures, but it is a great way to increase awareness of and establish a diagnosis of osteoporosis. There are several techniques for measuring BMD, but the gold standard is dual-energy X-ray absorptiometry (DEXA). Other methods of assessing bone mass include computerized tomography (CT) scans, ultrasound of the heel, and radiographs, but none of these are as optimal as DEXA for diagnosis and follow-up.

In addition to providing the most reliable measurement of bone density, DEXA requires less radiation exposure than a conventional radiograph or CT scan. Usually, DEXA is used to measure the density of both the hip and the lumbar spine. The hip is the preferred site for BMD testing, especially in women older than 60, because the spinal measurements can be unreliable. Although peripheral DEXA sites are accurate, they may be less useful because they may not correlate as well with fracture risk and BMD at the hip and spine. The guidelines for indications for BMD testing established by many reputable and independent organizations are as follows:

- ▸ Secondary causes of bone loss (e.g., steroid use, hyperparathyroidism)

- ▸ Radiological (X-ray) evidence of osteopenia (insufficient bone mineral density)

▶ All women 65 years and older (not only for a diagnosis, but also as a historical reference point for future comparisons)

▶ Younger postmenopausal women with fractures due to fragile bones since menopause, low body weight, or family history of spine or hip fracture

Results of BMD tests are reported as standard deviations—either a Z-score or a T-score. The Z-score is based on the standard deviation from the mean BMD of women in the same age group. The T-score is based on the mean peak BMD of a normal, young woman. The criteria established by WHO for the diagnosis of osteoporosis use T-scores: a score below −2.5 is associated with osteoporosis. The classification of osteopenia signifies a BMD that is between normal and osteoporosis.

Interpretation of Bone Mineral Density Scores

Status	T-score	Interpretation
Normal	Above −1	BMD within 1 SD of a young normal adult
Osteopenia	Between −1 and −2.5	BMD between 1 and 2.5 SD below a young normal adult
Osteoporosis	Below −2.5	BMD is 2.5 SD or more below a young normal adult

BMD = bone mineral density; SD = standard deviation.

FOSAMAX—WHAT IS THE REAL BENEFIT?

Merck's introduction of Fosamax coincided with the publication of the Fracture Intervention Trial, a study funded by Merck.[26] At first glance the claims made in Merck's advertisements for Fosamax were quite impressive: Merck claimed that, compared with a placebo, Fosamax reduced the rate of hip fractures by 50 percent. But if you take a closer look, the numbers do not seem so rosy. First of all, the women in the study were high-risk women who had a history of a fracture due to osteoporosis. Next, when you look at the absolute number of hip fractures that occurred during the four-year trial, the perspective changes dramatically. Only two out of 100 women in the placebo group had a hip fracture during the trial, compared with one woman out of 100 in the Fosamax group. In other words, 98 women out of 100 in the Fosamax group would have fared just as well on a placebo. It is true that for individuals who are at a very high risk, bisphosphonate therapy may offer some benefits; but I am not convinced that these benefits cannot be obtained even more effectively through nondrug measures. In fact, if you look at clinical studies done with vitamin D, calcium, and vitamin K$_2$ it appears that the natural approach is far superior.

Keep in mind that women at high risk are a much smaller group than the tens of millions of women identified by the expanded definition of low bone density. In fact, bisphosphonates are prescribed just as often for women with osteopenia (bone mineral density that is lower than normal, but not low enough to be classified as osteoporosis) as for women with osteoporosis, even though there is no correlation between osteopenia and the risk of a hip fracture. Bisphosphonates and Evista have shown no effectiveness in the treatment of osteopenia, and are not indicated for such treatment, despite considerable efforts by the drug companies to convince doctors otherwise.[27]

So why are doctors prescribing bisphosphonate or Evista (or both) for millions of women with osteopenia in the United States, when the research does not show any clear benefit? Obviously, the reasons are the fear that "low" bone density creates, the doctors' desire to do something, and the effective advertising and marketing of these drugs. It is little wonder that sales are so high. These drugs, however, are associated with significant side effects. Instead of relying on a drug to reduce the risk of osteoporosis and hip fracture, the more rational approach would be to focus on diet, lifestyle, and supplements.

SIDE EFFECTS OF BISPHOSPHONATES
AND EVISTA

Granted, my patient population may have been a bit skewed because the patients came to see me to help them get off their prescription drugs, but the patients I saw on bisphosphonates complained mightily about the side effects. In fact, I cannot recall anyone who really tolerated these drugs. Most of the side effects are mild: they include minor digestive disturbances such as heartburn, diarrhea, and flatulence; muscle and joint pain; headaches; and allergic reactions. However, early on the risk of severe damage to the esophagus was not known, and I did have a few patients who had suffered this serious side effect as well as more debilitating muscle pain. It is very important that anyone taking a bisphosphonate remain standing or seated upright for 45 to 60 minutes after taking the medication.

Bisphosphonates have also been associated with severe bone destruction (osteonecrosis) of the jaw. This side effect is most often seen in cancer patients or those undergoing dental work to eliminate potential sites of infection.

The most serious side effect for Evista and other SERMs is the formation of clots that can block veins or lodge in the lungs or heart. Though these side effects occur only in about one out of 100 patients treated with Evista, women treated with Evista are more than twice as likely to develop clot-related disease as women taking a placebo. More common side effects of Evista include difficult, burning, or painful urination; fever; increased rate of infections; leg cramps; skin rash; swelling of hands, ankles, or feet; and vaginal itching. Less common side effects include body aches and pains; congestion in the lungs; decreased vision or other changes in vision; diarrhea; difficulty in breathing; hoarseness; loss of appetite; nausea; trouble in swallowing; weakness.

A RATIONAL APPROACH TO OSTEOPOROSIS

Normal bone metabolism depends on an intricate interplay of many genetic, nutritional, lifestyle, and hormonal factors. A rational approach to osteoporosis involves reducing as many risk factors—that is, as many causes—as possible and at the same time incorporating as many causes; dietary and lifestyle factors that are extremely important in lowering the risk of osteoporosis. For example, smoking and excessive alcohol and caffeine increase the risk of developing osteoporosis, and regular exercise reduces the risk. In fact, numerous studies have clearly demonstrated that physical fitness is the major determinant of bone density. Physical exercise consisting of one hour of moderate activity three times a week has been shown to prevent bone loss and actually increase bone mass in postmenopausal women.[28]

Perhaps the most important dietary recommendation is to eat more green leafy vegetables and vegetables from the cabbage family, including broccoli, brussels sprouts, kale, collards, and mustard greens. These foods, as well as green tea, offer significant protection against osteoporosis. They are a rich source of a broad range of vitamins and minerals that are important to maintaining healthy bones, including calcium, vitamin K_1, and boron. Vitamin K_1 is the form of vitamin K that is found in plants. A function of vitamin K_1 is to convert inactive osteocalcin to its active form. Osteocalcin is an important protein in bone. Its role is to anchor calcium molecules and hold them in place within the bone. A higher intake of green leafy vegetables may be one of the key reasons that a vegetarian diet is associated with a lower risk of osteoporosis. Although bone mass in vegetarians does not differ significantly from that of omnivores in the third, fourth, and fifth decades of life, there are significant differences in later decades. These findings indicate that the decreased incidence of osteoporosis among vegetarians is due not to increased initial bone mass, but rather to decreased bone loss.[29, 30]

Here are some other important dietary considerations for preventing osteoporosis:

- Soft drinks containing phosphates (phosphoric acid) and sugar are strongly linked to osteoporosis and low bone density because they lead to lower calcium levels and higher phosphate levels in the blood.[31] When phosphate levels are high and calcium levels are low, calcium is pulled out of the bones. The phosphate content of soft drinks, such as Coca-Cola and Pepsi, is very high, and they contain virtually no calcium.

- ▶ Refined sugar also increases the loss of calcium from bone.[32] Regular consumption of refined sugar increases loss of calcium from the blood through the urine. Calcium is then pulled from the bones to maintain blood calcium levels, as foods containing refined sugar generally do not contain calcium.

- ▶ A diet high in salt or low in potassium also causes removal of calcium from bones and increases loss of calcium in the urine.[33] Therefore, avoid salt and eat more high-potassium foods, which include most fruits and vegetables.

- ▶ Adequate but not excessive protein is required for healthy bone.[34] Making a protein smoothie with 25 to 30 grams (g) of whey or soy protein powder is a great way to boost protein levels.

- ▶ Soy foods, such as tofu, soy milk, roasted soybeans and soy protein powders, may be beneficial in preventing osteoporosis. In several double-blind studies, taking 40 g of soy protein powder containing 90 milligrams (mg) of isoflavones increased bone mineral density of the spine and hips in postmenopausal women.[35, 36]

DOES MILK PREVENT OR CAUSE OSTEOPOROSIS?

Although numerous clinical studies have demonstrated that calcium and vitamin D supplementation can help prevent bone loss, the data are inconclusive with regard to any link between a high dietary calcium intake from milk and the prevention of osteoporosis and bone fractures. In fact, the current available data indicate that frequent consumption of milk actually increases the risk of osteoporosis. Reviewing the statistics from the Nurses' Health Study, which involved 77,761 women, researchers found that those who drank two or more glasses of milk per day had a 45 percent increased risk of hip fracture, compared with women who consumed one glass or less per week.[37] In other words, the more milk a woman consumed, the more likely she was to fracture a hip. This negative effect may turn out to be due to the vitamin A added to milk (at higher levels, vitamin A, but not beta-carotene, may interfere with bone formation). Interestingly, if you look at the rate of osteoporosis worldwide, it is considerably higher in countries where milk intake is highest.

Important Nutritional Supplements for Healthy Bones

▸ Calcium supplementation alone has shown little benefit in treating or preventing osteoporosis. But calcium supplementation combined with vitamin D can slow the rate of bone loss by as much as 30 percent, and it offers significant protection against hip fractures—cutting the risk by as much as half. The recommended dosage for calcium is 1,000 to 1,500 mg daily.[38, 39, 40]

▸ Vitamin D supplementation is associated with increased bone density, and studies that combined vitamin D with calcium produced better results than those that used either nutrient alone.[39, 40, 41, 42] Vitamin D supplementation is especially helpful for elderly people who don't get sufficient exposure to sunlight (which stimulates the body's manufacture of vitamin D). The recommended daily dose of vitamin D is 1,000 to 2,000 international units (IU).

▸ Magnesium supplementation is thought by some experts to be as important as calcium supplementation in the prevention and treatment of osteoporosis.[43, 44] Women with osteoporosis have more indicators of magnesium deficiency, such as lower bone magnesium content, than people without osteoporosis. The recommended dosage is 250 to 400 mg daily.

▸ Vitamin B_6, folic acid, and vitamin B_{12} are important in the conversion of the amino acid methionine to cysteine. If a person is deficient in these vitamins, there will be an increase in the level of homocysteine.

Homocysteine can act to damage cell structures and has been implicated in a variety of conditions, including atherosclerosis and osteoporosis.[45] Combinations of these vitamins will produce better results than any one of them alone. The recommended daily dosages are 15 to 25 mg for vitamin B_6, and 800 micrograms (μg) for folic acid and vitamin B_{12}.

▸ Calcium is not the only nutrient that is important for bone formation. Many trace minerals such as copper, manganese, zinc, and boron are also important. A deficiency in trace minerals can also predispose someone to osteoporosis. For example, boron is a trace mineral that has gained attention as a protective factor against osteoporosis. It appears that boron is required to activate certain hormones, including estrogen and vitamin D. In order to guarantee adequate boron levels, supplementing the diet with a daily dose of 3 to 5 mg of boron is recommended.[44, 46]

▸ Although vitamin K_1 from green leafy vegetables is important to healthy bone, vitamin K_2 supplements may have an even more powerful influence in women with existing osteoporosis. A number of clinical trials in Japan have shown that vitamin K_2 at high dosages (45 mg daily) can actually increase bone density and reduce hip fractures in postmenopausal women with osteoporosis when used in conjunction with calcium and vitamin D.[47, 48] In fact, the results from one study of 200 elderly female patients receiving either a placebo or 45 mg of vitamin K_2 (menatetrenone), 1,000 IU of vitamin D, and 600 mg of calcium showed that bone density increased by 2.3 percent in the treated group and decreased by 5.2 percent in the placebo group. Twenty-two patients in the untreated group sustained fractures (15 had hip fractures), but there were only three fractures (two hip fractures) in the group getting the vitamin therapy. That translates to a reduction of 87 percent in the risk of hip and other fractures in this high-risk group (compared with a placebo group), a reduction significantly better than that achieved with bisphosphonates.

A QUICK AND EASY WAY TO REDUCE
HEALTH CARE COSTS AND EXTEND LIFE

Considerable attention is focused on the need for increased levels of calcium, but most experts now agree that much greater attention should be focused on vitamin D. Its metabolic products not only stimulate calcium absorption but slow bone loss, increase bone formation, and reduce the risk of falling. It is estimated that by simply supplementing the diet with 1,000 to 1,200 mg of calcium and 800 to 1,000 IU of vitamin D more than half of all hip fractures could be prevented. The economic consequences of such a policy would be enormous: over a five-year period, more than 734,000 hip fractures could be avoided and more than $13.9 billion in health care costs could be saved. In addition, an analysis of studies with vitamin D showed that the participants who took vitamin D supplements had a 7 percent lower risk of death during the study period than those who did not.[49] Of course, this result is not surprising. It is now known that virtually every cell in our body has receptors for vitamin D and that vitamin D is not just a vitamin. It also performs very powerful hormonal activities and has protective effects against certain cancers (particularly cancer of the breast and prostate), autoimmune diseases such as multiple sclerosis and type 1 diabetes, and heart disease.[50] So, lack of vitamin D would affect far more than just our bones. Can you imagine the marketing that a drug company would put behind a drug that was shown to increase your chance of living longer? Sadly, this benefit of vitamin D has gone largely ignored because there is no financial reward for getting the word out.

A recent study published in the *American Journal of Clinical Nutrition* has added another major benefit for vitamin D and also provides an explanation for its promotion of longevity.[51] Vitamin D may slow aging by increasing the length of telomeres. A telomere is the section of a chromosome that shortens each time a cell replicates. The shorter the telomere gets, the more it affects gene expression. The result is cellular aging. In this study, scientists considered the effects of vitamin D on the length of telomeres in white blood cells of 2,160 women aged 18 to 79 years. The higher the vitamin D levels, the longer the telomere. In terms of the effect on aging, there was a five-year difference in telomere length in those with the highest levels of vitamin D compared with those with the lowest levels. Obesity, smoking, and lack of physical activity can shorten the telomere, but the researchers found that increasing vitamin D levels overcame these effects. What this five-year difference means is that a 70-year-old women with higher vitamin D levels would have a biological age of 65 years.

Troubling Statistics on Vitamin D Deficiency

40 percent of the U.S. population are deficient in vitamin D.

42 percent of African-American women of childbearing age are deficient in vitamin D.

48 percent of girls (nine to 11 years old are deficient in vitamin D.

60 percent of all hospital patients are deficient in vitamin D.

76 percent of pregnant women are severely deficient in vitamin D.

80 percent of nursing home patients are deficient in vitamin D.

HOW TO INCREASE YOUR VITAMIN D LEVELS

Since vitamin D can be produced in our bodies by the action of sunlight on the skin, many experts consider it more a hormone than a vitamin. Sunlight changes a compound (7-dehydrocholesterol) in the skin into vitamin D_3 (cholecalciferol). It is generally thought that as little as 15 minutes of direct sunlight on the skin can significantly raise vitamin D levels, but recent research has challenged this conventional wisdom. For example, from the latitude of San Francisco northward—or from Buenos Aires southward—for three to six months of the year, no amount of exposure will generate substantial vitamin D in even the palest skin.[52]

To ensure adequate vitamin D levels, supplementation is warranted, especially for those who live in a high latitude or who get little direct sunlight. There are two major dietary forms of vitamin D: vitamin D_2 (ergocalciferol) and vitamin D_3 (cholecalciferol). Vitamin D_2 is the form most often added to milk and other foods, as well as the form most often used in nutritional supplements. Vitamin D_3 in nutritional supplements is most often derived from fish liver oil or lanolin. Both D_2 and D_3 are capable of being converted to active vitamin D in the body. Very few foods naturally contain vitamin D or are fortified. Fish such as wild salmon (360 IU per 3.5-ounce serving), mackerel, and sardines are good sources of vitamin D_3. Fortified foods including milk (100 IU per 8-ounce serving), orange juice (100 IU per 8-ounce serving), and some breads and cereals provide D_2. The reason I have specified wild salmon is that the vitamin D content of farmed salmon is 75 percent less than that of wild caught salmon from Alaska.[52]

Recently, most experts have been recommending a daily intake of 800 to 1,000 IU of vitamin D. Although vitamin D conceivably has the potential to cause toxicity, dosages in the range of 800 to 2,000 IU per day are now recognized as being safe levels.[53]

The drugs cholestyramine (Questran), colestipol (Colestid), phenytoin (Dilantin), and phenobarbital, and mineral oil, all interfere with the absorption or metabolism (or both) of vitamin D. So, you will need to take vitamin D at the higher recommended dosage, 2,000 IU daily. The same is true if you are taking corticosteroids such as prednisone, because they increase the need for vitamin D. Vitamin D supplementation must be used with caution if you are taking digoxin (Lanoxin®) and thiazide diuretics: in that case, do not take more than 400 to 800 IU of vitamin D daily without consulting your physician.

FINAL COMMENTS

I think it makes sense for women to have a baseline test of bone density. Though these tests are being abused—in the sense that they simply serve to justify prescribing a drug—they do provide information that is valuable in bolstering bone health through diet, lifestyle, and nutritional supplements. Many medical associations recommend having this baseline test done at age 65, but my feeling is that it makes even more sense when women are in their thirties and forties, because the natural approach to building bone is even more effective then. The test is useful for men only if there is some factor that may predispose them to osteoporosis, such as long-term use of prednisone or another corticosteroid.

The test assesses how much bone mass you currently have. It will tell you whether you need to make an even more serious effort to maintain your bone. Information from the test can be used in later years to measure the rate of bone loss. Of course, a bone density test may also tell you that you already have osteoporosis.

Once you know your current bone density, the next step is to monitor how fast your bones are breaking down. The easiest way to do this is to measure the products of bone loss in the urine. The test I recommend is the Osteomark-NTX. It can provide valuable information on the rate of bone breakdown, and you should ask your doctor for it.

7

EXPLOITING THE
CHOLESTEROL MYTH

"For every complicated problem there is a solution that
is simple, direct, understandable and wrong."
—H. L. Mencken

THE CHOLESTEROL-LOWERING STATIN DRUGS are another example of how the drug industry uses its muscle to peddle a product. These drugs are sold primarily on the premise that they will save lives by lowering cholesterol levels, but in reality they have not convincingly demonstrated an ability to extend life in women, and they produce very little effect in men who show no clinical evidence of heart disease. Also, statins involve a significant risk of serious side effects. It is a one-sided situation: the drugs provide no real benefit to the person taking them, but they are a very important source of revenue for the drug companies. Annual sales of these drugs now exceed $25 billion. They generate huge profits for the drug companies. The statin "empire" is perhaps the greatest accomplishment of the modern drug industry, and this is an achievement the drug companies and doctors should be ashamed of.

The only reason we are so fixated on cholesterol is the influence of the pharmaceutical industry. It is very interesting to note that more than half the people who die of a heart attack or a stroke have low to normal cholesterol levels. How do the drug companies and the government respond to this fact? They simply recommend making the suggested target cholesterol levels even lower, thereby effectively casting an even wider net for potential customers. Their goal is to turn all of us into patients hooked on statins. It is also very interesting that six of the nine expert members of the government panel that drafted the new cholesterol guidelines had either received grants from or were paid consulting or speakers' fees by the companies that make some of the most popular statin drugs. There may be a conflict of interest here, but in any case these new guidelines should dramatically increase the number of patients on statin drugs. Keep in mind that statins are already the biggest moneymakers in the drug industry.

Although high cholesterol levels are associated with an increased risk of a heart attack or stroke, the relationship of cholesterol to these cardiovascular diseases (CVDs) is much more complex than the drug companies and many doctors portray it. According to conventional wisdom, lowering cholesterol with statin drugs should decrease the risk of CVD. But except for those taking statins because of a prior heart attack or another significant risk factor, the science simply does not support this assumption. As noted by the nineteenth-century scientist Thomas Huxley, "The great tragedy of science is the slaying of a beautiful hypothesis by an ugly fact."

Top Five Statin Drug Sales in 2005

1. Lipitor (Pfizer)—$12.2 billion

2. Zocor (Merck)—$4.4 billion

3. Vytorin (Merck and Schering-Plough—$2.4 billion

4. Pravachol (Bristol-Myers Squib)—$2.3 billion

5. Crestor (Astra-Zeneca)—$1.3 billion

WHAT IS HEART DISEASE?

"Heart disease" and "cardiovascular disease" (or CVD) refer to many diseases of or injuries to the cardiovascular system, which includes the heart, the blood vessels of the heart (coronary arteries), and the system of blood vessels—veins and arteries—throughout the body and within the brain. By far the biggest contributor to CVD is atherosclerosis—hardening of the artery walls due to a buildup of plaque containing cholesterol, fatty material, and cellular debris. Normally your arteries are very flexible, like a rubber tube. Plaque causes them to become stiff and can even block blood flow. Arterial plaque can also lead to the formation of blood clots—thickened clumps of blood that form when disk-shaped cells called platelets collect at the site of blood vessel damage. If a piece of the plaque or clot breaks off, it will eventually circulate into a vessel that is too small to allow it to pass. As a result, blood flow to that part of the body stops, and a nearby organ or tissue can die. A heart attack (also called a myocardial infarction) occurs when something blocks the flow of blood to the heart—it can be a clot, a spasm of a coronary artery, or an accumulation of plaque. Likewise, a stroke occurs when the blood flow to the brain is interrupted by a clot, the buildup of plaque, or the bursting of a vessel.

Of the CVDs, heart attacks and strokes are the leading causes of death. In fact, about 2,400 people die of a heart attack or stroke each day in the United States. That's approximately one death every 36 seconds; in other words, in the time it will probably take you to finish reading this chapter, more than 30 people will have died of these two CVDs. This number is staggering to contemplate—think of all the hardship and pain this cause of premature death produces for millions of people each year. Despite the enormous amounts of money being spent to thwart CVD, including the fixation on lowering cholesterol, lives continue to be lost.

High cholesterol levels are an important risk factor to address, but more than 200 other risk factors have been identified for heart disease. Other risk factors considered major are smoking, diabetes, high blood pressure, obesity, and lack of physical activity. There are also some very important dietary and lifestyle factors that the drug companies are not going to tell you about and your doctor may not know about. You absolutely must address these factors if you want to reduce your risk of having a heart attack or stroke. The fixation on cholesterol by the drug companies and doctors at the expense of natural approaches is one of the greatest medical injustices of all time.

Some Important Facts about Cardiovascular Disease (CVD):

▸ Mortality data show that CVD was the underlying cause of death in one out of every 2.8 deaths in the United States in 2004.

▸ In every year since 1900 (except 1918), CVD accounted for more deaths than any other single cause or group of causes in the United States. (Note: In 1918, Spanish influenza was the number one cause of death.)

▸ Nearly 2,400 Americans die of CVD each day, an average of 1 death every 36 seconds.

▸ CVD claims more lives each year than the following causes combined: cancer, chronic lower respiratory diseases, accidents, and diabetes mellitus.

▸ The probability at birth of eventually dying from CVD is 47 percent, and the probability of dying from cancer is 22 percent. Additional probabilities are 3 percent for accidents, 2 percent for diabetes, and 0.7 percent for HIV-AIDS.

▸ If all major forms of CVD were eliminated, life expectancy would rise by almost seven years. If all forms of cancer were eliminated, it would rise by three years.

A CLOSER LOOK AT CHOLESTEROL

Though vilified, cholesterol is actually one of the most important substances in the human body. Almost 80 percent of all circulating cholesterol is manufactured in the liver; only 20 percent comes from dietary sources. Cholesterol is found in the bloodstream and in virtually every cell of the body. The functions of cholesterol are many; here is a short list of the impressive features of this presumed culprit.

1. Cholesterol is used to form cell membranes; without it, cells lose their ability to function properly.

2. Cholesterol is a building block for vitamin D and for many hormones, including cortisol, testosterone, progesterone, and estrogens.

3. Cholesterol is vital for proper neurological function, playing a role in memory and uptake of hormones in the brain.

Cholesterol travels from the liver and into your circulation by hitching a ride on protein molecules such as low-density lipoprotein (LDL), often called "bad" cholesterol. It is carried away from tissues and back to the liver aboard high-density lipoprotein (HDL): ("good" or "protective" cholesterol).

The more LDL you have, the more cholesterol is in circulation, and the greater your risk of heart disease. Currently, experts recommend that your total blood cholesterol level should be less than 200 milligrams per deciliter (mg/dL). The LDL level should be less than 160 mg/dL. If you have had a heart attack, are a smoker, have a significant family history of CVD, or have diabetes, then it is recommended that you get the LDL below 100 mg/dL. But keep in mind that other factors need to be taken into consideration. For example, the level of HDL should be greater than 50 mg/dL. The level of HDL is considerably more important than LDL, but since statins do not affect this measurement, most doctors do not make a big deal about it. It is estimated that for every 1 percent drop in LDL levels, there's a 2 percent drop in the risk of heart attack. By the same token, for every 1 percent increase in HDL, the risk of heart attack drops 3 or 4 percent. In the famous Framingham study, no patients had a heart attack if their HDL was greater than 75 mg/dL irrespective of how high their LDL was.

The ratio of total cholesterol to HDL and the ratio of LDL to HDL are clues that indicate whether cholesterol is being deposited in tissues or is being broken down and excreted. The ratio of total cholesterol to HDL should be no higher than 4.2, and the ratio of LDL to HDL ratio should be no higher than 2.5.

Actually, there's a form of LDL that's even worse: it's called lipoprotein (a), or Lp(a). It looks like LDL, but it has an additional molecule of an adhesive protein, apolipoprotein. That protein makes the molecule much more likely to stick to the artery walls. New research suggests that high

Understanding Risk Factors

Heart disease and strokes are often referred to as silent killers because in many cases the first symptom or sign is a fatal event. The good news about CVD is that it is highly preventable if as many risk factors as possible are eliminated. The major risk factors are generally considered to be:

- Smoking
- Elevated blood cholesterol levels
- High blood pressure
- Diabetes
- Obesity
- Physical inactivity

If two or more of these major factors apply to you, your risk increases significantly. For example, if you smoke, have high cholesterol, and have high blood pressure, you are more than 700 times likelier to have heart disease—and you will probably die 20 to 30 years sooner—than someone without any of these factors.

The More Risk Factors, the Greater the Risk

CONDITION	INCREASED RISK OF HEART DISEASE
Presence of 1 major risk factor	30%
High cholesterol + high blood pressure	300%
High cholesterol + smoking	350%
High blood pressure + smoking	350%
Smoking + high blood pressure + high cholesterol	720%

In addition to these widely acknowledged major risk factors, there are numerous other factors that have been shown in many cases to be more significant than the presumably major ones. Here are some of the most important of these other risk factors:

- ► Low levels of omega-3 fatty acids
- ► Elevations of markers of silent inflammation, such as C-reactive protein (CRP) and fibrinogen.
- ► Low dietary antioxidant status
- ► Low levels of magnesium and potassium
- ► Low levels of folic acid, leading to elevations in homocysteine
- ► Type A personality

Lp(a) levels constitute a separate risk factor for heart attack. For example, it appears that high Lp(a) levels are 10 times more likely to cause heart disease than high LDL levels; Lp(a) levels lower than 20 mg/dL are associated with low risk of heart disease; levels between 20 and 40 mg/dL pose a moderate risk; and levels higher than 40 mg/dL are considered extremely risky.

THE STATIN "EMPIRE"

The statin drug "empire" consists of the popular cholesterol-lowering drugs, such as Crestor (rosuvastatin), Lipitor (atorvastatin), Zocor (simvastatin), Mevacor (lovastatin), and Pravachol (provastatin); and similar drugs that lower cholesterol by inhibiting an enzyme in the liver (HMG-CoA reductase) that manufactures cholesterol. As noted earlier, annual sales of these drugs now exceed $25 billion. Millions of prescriptions are filled yearly in the hope of reducing the risk of developing heart disease. But, the results of detailed studies indicate that the majority of people on statin drugs are achieving no real benefit. In fact, relying on these drugs and not focusing on effectively reducing the risk of heart disease through diet, lifestyle, and proper nutritional supplementation is costing many people their lives. In addition, although drug companies and many doctors state that statins are so safe and effective that they should be placed in drinking water, they are really very expensive medicines, provide very limited benefit, and involve a considerable risk of side effects. Side effects noted with statins include:

- Liver problems and elevated liver function.

- Interference with the manufacture of coenzyme Q10—a substance responsible for energy production within the body.

- Rhabdomyolysis—a breaking down of muscle tissue, which can prove fatal.

- Nerve damage is a real risk. The chance of nerve damage is 26 times higher for statin users than for people who do not take statins.

- Impaired mental functions can occur in some patients after prolonged use.

- Possible increased risk of cancer and heart failure after long-term use.

Numerous long-term studies have shown quite convincingly that for people with existing CVD or diabetes, statins do produce some benefit in reducing deaths due to a heart attack, but the overall effect on life expectancy remains somewhat controversial. For example, in the large Heart Protection Study men with CVD who took a statin for five years reduced their chance of death only slightly: from 15 percent to 13 percent.[1] Moreover, a reduced rate of heart attacks and strokes may be offset by an increase in other causes of death (e.g., possibly cancer) during the study period.

The larger issue is whether statins have any benefit for people with no evidence of CVD. About 75 percent of the prescriptions for statins are written for people with no clinical evidence of CVD. But whereas there is some evidence (though not all very impressive evidence) of prevention against a second heart attack (secondary prevention), the benefit of statins in preventing a first heart attack or stroke (primary prevention) has not been proved to any sufficient standard. So, prescribing statins for primary prevention of death due to CVD is not consistent with scientific studies. Several large evaluations of studies of people with no history of a heart attack or stroke who took statin drugs and lowered their cholesterol have shown they did not live any longer than the people in the placebo groups.[2, 3, 4] Occasionally, there is a positive study with a statin drug, showing some reduction of mortality (of course, funded by a drug company), but the effect noted pales in comparison with the effect of dietary and lifestyle interventions. For example, one study reported in the *New England Journal of Medicine* looked at the activity level and health of retired men in Honolulu between the ages of 61 and 81.[5] These men were followed for more than 10 years and divided into two groups: one group walked less than one mile per day; the other group walked more than two miles per day. The group that walked more than two miles per day had almost 50 percent fewer deaths during that period than those who walked less than one mile per day. Interesting—a drug-free plan that cost nothing had a better effect on mortality during the period studied than the high-priced cholesterol-lowering drugs.

Is a Siesta More Effective Than a Statin Drug?

An afternoon nap (a siesta) is common in populations with low rates of death from heart attacks. To study the benefit of a siesta for heart health, researchers selected subjects carefully to prevent variables such as physical activity and diet from interfering with a statistical analysis. The analysis was conducted on results from the Greek European Prospective Investigation into Cancer and Nutrition (EPIC) study, involving 23,681 individuals who at enrollment had no history of coronary heart disease, stroke, or cancer and provided complete information on frequency and duration of midday napping.[6] These subjects were followed up for an average of nearly 6.5 years. The results were astounding. People who took a siesta of any frequency or duration had a 34 percent reduced rate of having a heart attack. Further analysis showed that occasional napping produced a 12 percent lower coronary mortality rate, and those who napped regularly had a 37 percent lower coronary mortality. These results are far superior to the results demonstrated with statin drugs in the primary prevention of CVD and raises the question, "Is taking a nap more effective in preventing a heart attack than taking a statin?" The answer appears to be yes.

A CLOSER LOOK AT HOW STATINS WORK

Statins work by blocking an enzyme (HMG-CoA reductase) that produces a compound (mevalonate) that is the direct precursor to cholesterol. The problem is that statins inhibit the production not only of cholesterol but also of many other bodily substances that have important biochemical functions. These include coenzyme Q10 and dolichols.

Coenzyme Q10 (CoQ10) is a critical component in the manufacture of ATP—the energy currency of our cells. Basically, the role of CoQ10 in the our cells is similar to the role of a spark plug in a car engine. Just as the car cannot function without that initial spark, the cell cannot function without CoQ10. Although the body makes some of its own CoQ10, considerable research shows significant benefits with supplementation. Also, people with any sort of heart disease, including high cholesterol levels and high blood pressure, and people taking cholesterol-lowering drugs are known to have low CoQ10 levels.

Since statin drugs reduce the production of CoQ10, they would obviously have some serious consequences, because organs such as the heart, liver, and brain require large amounts of CoQ10 to function properly, as do the muscles. The research seems to support this observation: the serious side effects due to statin drugs appear to be related to lowering CoQ10 levels.[7, 8] In addition, deaths attributed to heart failure have nearly doubled since 1989—an interesting fact because statins first reached the market in a big way in 1988. If you are taking a statin drug, you definitely need supplemental CoQ10 at a dosage of 100 to 200 mg daily. Choose soft gel capsules with rice bran oil for maximum absorption.

Dolichols are less talked about, but they are another component of the cholesterol pathway whose production is also inhibited by statin drugs. Like CoQ10, dolichols are very important in human biology. One of their functions is to help direct proteins to targeted cells. In other words, when your liver or other tissue makes certain proteins, those proteins need to be delivered to the specific destinations; dolichols make that possible. Since statin drugs can reduce the amount of dolichols in circulation, they may bring

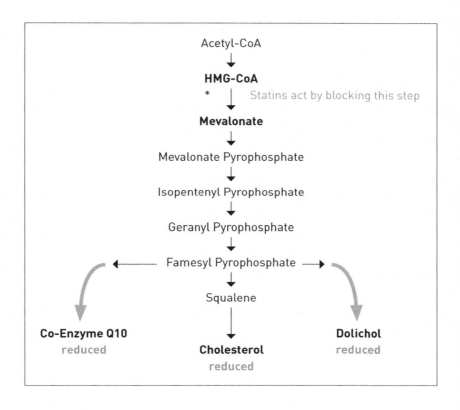

chaos to our bodily processes. A good analogy would be a large city with no street signs or addresses; mail would never be delivered and outsiders could never find their destinations.

I stressed in Chapter 5 that relieving symptoms is often a path to bad medicine. What is happening here is tunnel vision. To focus solely on lowering cholesterol with statins is to ignore the fact that we are inhibiting a natural process in the body. Remember that cholesterol is an important substance in the body, involved in hormone production, digestion, and the manufacturing of cell membranes. Could inhibiting it have other consequences that are even more dangerous than elevated cholesterol levels? The answer to this question seems buried in the confusing science of statins and their serious consequences.

AN HONEST APPRAISAL OF THE BENEFITS
OF STATINS IN PRIMARY PREVENTION

The drug companies and most doctors want us to believe that since statins lower cholesterol, they most assuredly reduce the risk of heart attacks and strokes in people who do not have CVD. As with most cases of conventional wisdom, this link is convenient but the scientific data simply show otherwise. There is no question that in population studies, lower levels of cholesterol are correlated with a reduced number of deaths due to CVD. But lowering cholesterol levels with statins has not been proved to reduce this risk or increase life expectancy in subjects without CVD, despite a considerable effort by the drug companies. A careful review of studies of the major statin drugs involving subjects without clinical evidence of CVD shows that there were no significant differences in mortality from CVD between people who took cholesterol-lowering agents and those who took a placebo. Pooled data from eight randomized trials that compared statins with a placebo in primary prevention of mortality from CVD showed that such mortality was not reduced by statins.[8] For example:

▸ Statins did not reduce total heart attacks or strokes in 10,990 women in the primary prevention trials.[9]

▸ In 3,239 men and women older than 69 years, statins did not reduce total heart attacks or strokes.[10]

▸ In 10,355 patients with high blood pressure who were chosen at random to receive a placebo or drug therapy using a statin (Pravastatin, 40 mg/day), there was no significant difference in the rate of death, heart disease, and heart attack.[11]

▸ In a study involving 47,294 patients without CVD, researchers gave participants either 40 mg of simvastatin or a placebo. There was no correlation between lowered LDL cholesterol and death rate during the study.[12]

The consensus among most medical experts not aligned with or supported by the drug companies is that statins should not be prescribed for the primary prevention of CVD mortality in women of any age or for men older than 69 years. Keep in mind that although statins have been shown to provide a statistical benefit in reducing CVD mortality in high-risk men aged 30 to 69 years, about 50 percent need to be treated for a minimum of five years to prevent one stroke or heart attack. Obviously, relying on statin drugs in lieu of important dietary, lifestyle, and nutritional supplement approaches does not make very much sense.

Because CVD is a multifactorial issue, any attempt to simplify it by addressing only one risk factor is doomed to fail. Simply stated, there are more important things to consider than the level of LDL cholesterol. The whole premise of reducing LDL cholesterol levels with statins is the mistaken belief that this will reduce the buildup of arterial plaque, but researchers at Beth Israel Medical Center in New York City demonstrated the real reason statins do not work.[13] They examined the buildup of coronary plaque in patients who took statins at either a dosage of more than 80 mg/day or a dosage of less than 80 mg/day. At the beginning of the study the coronary arterial plaque of all the patients was measured by electron beam tomography. At the end of the 12-month study, cholesterol levels and coronary plaque were again measured. Although both groups were successful in lowering their cholesterol, the reduction didn't appear to have nay statistical effect on the buildup of plaque. In other words, the buildup of plaque (which is the reason why doctors try to lower cholesterol) didn't appear to be related to cholesterol levels. Again, there are other factors involved in the process of atherosclerosis that are significantly more important than lowering cholesterol, but are largely ignored because they do not involve drug therapy.

DIET VERSUS STATINS

Dietary measures alone are often extremely effective in lowering cholesterol levels. For example, in one interesting study[14] the participants were randomly assigned to receive one of three interventions on an outpatient basis

for one month: (1) a diet low in saturated fat; (2) the same diet plus lovastatin, 20 mg/day; or (3) a diet high in plant sterols, soy protein, soluble dietary
fiber, and almonds. The control group, statin group, and "dietary portfolio"
group had average decreases in LDL cholesterol of 8 percent, 30.9 percent,
and 28.6 percent, respectively. These results indicate that incorporating several dietary components known to lower cholesterol levels produced results
comparable to those obtained with a statin drug.

Here are the key dietary recommendations to reduce the risk of atherosclerosis:

▸ Reduce the amount of saturated fat, trans fatty acids, cholesterol, and
total fat in your diet by eating fewer animal products and more plant
foods.

▸ Increase your intake of omega-3 oils by eating flaxseed oil, walnuts,
and small amounts of cold-water fish. There is considerable evidence
that people who consume a diet rich in omega-3 oils from either fish
or vegetable sources have a significantly reduced risk of developing
atherosclerosis. Atherosclerosis is associated with a deficiency in
omega-3 oils.

▸ Increase your intake of heart-healthy monounsaturated fats by eating
more nuts and seeds—including almonds, Brazil nuts, coconut,
hazelnuts, macadamia nuts, pecans, pine nuts, pistachios, sesame
seeds, and sunflower seeds—and using a monounsaturated oil, such as
olive or canola oil, for cooking. Keep intake moderate, however,
because these are high-calorie foods. Limit nuts and seeds to no more
than ¼ cup daily and monounsaturated oil to 2 tablespoons.

▸ Eat five or more servings daily of a combination of vegetables and
fruits, especially green, orange, and yellow vegetables; dark-colored
berries; and citrus fruits. Antioxidant compounds in these plant foods,
such as carotenes, flavonoids, selenium, vitamin E, and vitamin C, are
important in protecting against the development of atherosclerosis.
These foods are also rich in B vitamins that can help lower
homocysteine levels.

▶ Increase your intake of fiber. A diet high in fiber has been shown to protect against atherosclerosis. Dietary fiber, particularly the soluble fiber found in legumes, fruit, and vegetables, is effective in lowering cholesterol levels.

▶ Limit your intake of refined carbohydrates (sugar and refined grains). Sugar and other refined carbohydrates are a significant factor in the development of atherosclerosis. Sugar elevates levels of the hormone insulin. Elevated insulin levels, in turn, are associated with increased cholesterol and triglycerides, higher blood pressure, and risk of death from cardiovascular disease.

One diet that appears to represent a way of eating that provides significant protection against heart disease is the traditional "Mediterranean diet." This term has a specific meaning; it does not mean simply Italian food. The Mediterranean diet reflects food patterns typical of Crete, parts of the rest of Greece, and southern Italy in the early 1960s. The traditional Mediterranean diet has shown tremendous benefits in fighting heart disease and cancer, as well as diabetes.[15, 16, 17] It has the following characteristics:

▶ It centers on an abundance of plant food, including fruit, vegetables, breads, pasta, potatoes, beans, nuts, and seeds.

▶ Foods are minimally processed and there is a focus on seasonal, fresh, and locally grown foods.

▶ Fresh fruit is the typical daily dessert. Sweets containing concentrated sugars or honey are consumed a few times per week at the most.

▶ Low-fat dairy products, principally cheese and yogurt, are consumed daily in low to moderate amounts.

▶ Fish is consumed on a regular basis.

▶ Poultry and eggs are consumed in moderate amounts, about one to four times weekly, or not at all.

▶ Red meat is consumed in small amounts, and infrequently.

▶ Olive oil is the principal source of fat.

▶ Wine is consumed in low to moderate amounts, normally with meals.

Two components of the Mediterranean diet that have received a lot of attention are red wine and olive oil. Red wine is thought to be responsible for the "French paradox"—a term referring to the fact that the French consume more saturated fat than Americans yet have a lower incidence of heart disease. The explanation is that the flavonoids in red wine protect against oxidative damage to the arteries from LDL cholesterol.

Olive oil contains a heart-protective monounsaturated fatty acid, oleic acid. It also contains several antioxidant agents that prevent circulating LDL cholesterol from becoming damaged and then subsequently damaging the arteries. Olive oil lowers harmful LDL cholesterol and increases the level of protective HDL cholesterol. It has also been proved to lower elevated blood triglycerides though in this regard it is not as effective as fish oils.

C-Reactive Protein and Diet

Silent inflammation is an important factor in the buildup of atherosclerotic plaque. To measure the degree of inflammation, physicians determine the level of C-reactive protein (CRP) in the blood. This is one of the acute phase proteins that increase during systemic inflammation. Most studies show that the higher the CRP level, the higher the risk of heart attack, even in people with low LDL cholesterol.

If the CRP level is lower than 1.0 milligrams per liter (mg/L), there is a low risk of developing cardiovascular disease. If CRP is between 1.0 and 3.0 mg/L, there is an average risk. If CRP is higher than 3.0 mg/L, there is a high risk.

Dietary interventions alone have been shown to lower CRP levels. In particular, the Mediterranean diet can be quite effective in lowering CRP levels to normal.[17]

REDISCOVERING NIACIN

One of the first cholesterol-lowering agents was a B vitamin, niacin. The research on the safety and effectiveness of niacin is exceptional and in many respects far superior to that of the statin drugs. Niacin has been shown to reduce LDL cholesterol, Lp(a) lipoprotein, triglyceride, and fibrinogen while simultaneously increasing HDL cholesterol. Most important, in the famous Coronary Drug Project (CDP), niacin was found to reduce the five-year incidence of heart attacks by 27 percent. And here is something that is very interesting; at the 15-year follow-up, nearly nine years after the trial was completed, all-cause mortality was 11 percent lower for the patients who took niacin than for those who took a placebo.[18, 19]

Despite the fact that niacin has demonstrated better overall results than statins in reducing risk factors for coronary heart disease, physicians are often reluctant to recommend niacin except in the form of the time-released prescription product Niaspan. The reason is a widespread perception by doctors that over-the-counter regular niacin is difficult to work with because of a bothersome flushing of the skin—like a prickly heat rash—which typically occurs 20 to 30 minutes after the niacin is taken and disappears in about 20 to 30 minutes more. Other occasional side effects of niacin include gastric irritation, nausea, and liver damage.

One main reason why niacin is not recommended more by doctors is that it is a widely available generic agent available over the counter in health food stores and drugstores, so no pharmaceutical company stands to enjoy the huge profits that the other lipid-lowering agents have generated. As a result, niacin does not get the intensive advertising that the statin drugs have been given. Despite the advantages of niacin over other lipid-lowering drugs, the prescription form, Niaspan, accounts for less than 10 percent of all cholesterol-lowering prescriptions.

Several studies have compared niacin with standard lipid-lowering drugs, including the statin drugs. These studies have shown significant advantages for niacin. For example, in one 26-week study patients were randomly assigned to receive treatment with either lovastatin (Mevacor) or niacin.[20] The results indicated that although lovastatin produced a greater reduction in LDL cholesterol (32 percent versus 23 percent), niacin produced better overall results. The percentage increase in HDL cholesterol, a more significant indicator for coronary heart disease, was dramatically in favor of niacin (33 percent versus 7 percent). Equally impressive was the percentage decrease in Lp(a) with niacin: niacin produced a 35 percent reduction in Lp(a) lipoprotein levels, whereas lovastatin did not have any effect. Other studies have shown that niacin can lower Lp(a) levels by an average of 38 percent.

In another study, a 3,000-mg dose of niacin was compared with 80 mg of atorvastatin.[21] The patients selected had abnormal particle size of LDL in that the LDL molecules were small and dense—such molecules are considerably more damaging to the arteries than larger, less dense LDL. The patients selected also had low levels (less than 40 percent) of a specific fraction of HDL associated with a greater protective effect than HDL alone. Although atorvastatin reduced total LDL cholesterol substantially more than niacin did, niacin was more effective than atorvastatin in increasing LDL particle size and raising HDL and HDL2.

Effect of Atorvastatin (Lipitor) and Niacin on Lipid Profiles

Lipid Measurement	ATORVASTATIN Before	ATORVASTATIN After	NIACIN Before	NIACIN After	ATORVASTATIN + NIACIN Before	ATORVASTATIN + NIACIN After
Total LDL (mg/dL)	110	56	111	89	123	55
LDL peak diameter	251	256	253	263	250	263
Lipoprotein (a) (mg/dL)	45	44	37	23	54	35
HDL (mg/dL)	42	43	38	54	38	54
HDL2 (%)	30	42	29	43	32	37
Triglycerides (mg/dL)	186	100	194	108	235	73

Because taking niacin at higher dosages (e.g., 3,000 mg or more daily) can impair glucose tolerance, many physicians have avoided prescribing niacin therapy for diabetics, but newer studies with slightly lower dosages of niacin (1,000 to 2,000 mg daily) have not shown any adverse effects on blood sugar regulation. For example, during a 16-week double-blind, placebo-controlled trial, 148 patients with type 2 diabetes were assigned at random to take a placebo or 1,000 or 1,500 mg/day of niacin; in the groups taking niacin, there was no significant loss of control over blood sugar and the favorable effects on blood lipids were still apparent.[22] Other studies have shown that niacin actually improves the control of blood sugar.[23] All told, niacin appears to be a very important recommendation for people with type 2 diabetes, as the most common blood lipid abnormalities in these patients are elevated triglyceride levels, decreased HDL cholesterol levels, and a preponderance of smaller, denser LDL particles. Niacin has been shown to address all these conditions much more significantly than the statins or other lipid-lowering drugs.

For Secondary Prevention of a Heart Attack, Add Niacin to a Statin

The dominant approach to reducing mortality from heart disease is the use of statins alone, but this approach is not really very effective at reducing death rates. The focus is almost entirely on reducing LDL cholesterol, but most patients with coronary heart disease also have low levels of HDL cholesterol and elevated triglycerides. The statins do not affect these blood lipids, but niacin does. When niacin is added to statin therapy, the results are outstanding. The HDL Atherosclerosis Treatment Study showed a 60 to 90 percent reduction of major coronary events when niacin was added to statin therapy.[24] In addition, combination treatment led to angiographic regression of coronary artery plaque, another benefit not seen with therapy involving only statins.

To reduce skin flushing as a side effect of niacin, you can use some of the newer time-released formulas, including the prescription version, Niaspan; or you can take regular over-the-counter niacin just before going to bed. Most people sleep right through the flushing reaction. Taking cholesterol-lowering agents at night is best in any case, because most of the cholesterol manufactured by the liver is produced at night. Another approach to reducing flushing is to use inositol hexaniacinate. This form of niacin has long been used in Europe to lower cholesterol levels and also to improve blood flow in intermittent claudication—a peripheral vascular disease that is quite common in diabetics. Inositol hexaniacinate has slightly better clinical results than standard niacin, and it is much better tolerated, in terms of both flushing and—more important—long-term side effects. If you start out with inositol hexaniacinate and it does not work, try regular niacin. Our experience is that some people will respond only to regular niacin.

If regular niacin or inositol hexaniacinate is being used, start with a dose of 500 mg at night before going to bed for one week. Increase the dosage to 1,000 mg the next week and to 1,500 mg the following week. Stay at 1,500 mg for two months before checking the response. Then, the dosage can be adjusted up or down, depending on the response. If you are using a time-release niacin product, such as Niaspan, start out at the full dosage of 1,500 mg at night.

Regardless of the form of niacin being used, I strongly recommend periodic checking (at a minimum of every 3 months the first year and once yearly thereafter) of cholesterol and liver enzymes.

ANOTHER NATURAL ALTERNATIVE TO STATINS

A few years ago, a friend asked me if there were any natural alternatives to the statin drug Lipitor. His physician had prescribed Lipitor after a routine yearly physical showed that his cholesterol level was 294 mg/dL and his "bad" LDL cholesterol level was 195 mg/dL. I told him there are many choices, but I wanted him to try a new product on the market—a combination of cholesterol-lowering plant sterols with Sytrinol (a special flavonoid from citrus peels). The research on Sytrinol is extremely impressive, and I was looking for a test subject, so I asked him to take three capsules in the morning and three capsules at night, providing a daily intake of 1,200 of the plant sterols and 450 mg of Sytrinol. His repeat blood test two months later showed that his total cholesterol had dropped to 190 mg/dL and his LDL was now 105 mg/dL. Both numbers are outstanding, representing a drop of more than 30 percent for total cholesterol and roughly 45 percent for LDL. Fantastic! It was just the response that I had hoped for.

Combining plant sterols with Sytrinol provides a comprehensive formula that addresses all facets of elevated blood lipids including high cholesterol, high LDL, and high triglycerides. Sytrinol also has a significant anti-inflammatory effect; this is important, because chronic inflammation has been shown to be a risk factor for heart attack. Recently, Sytrinol was shown to enhance insulin sensitivity. In total, all these effects make this natural heart health formula an ideal choice for anyone wishing to maintain a healthy lipid profile and reduce the risk of having a heart attack or stroke.

Clinical results have shown that Sytrinol has effects very similar to those of statin drugs, but without side effects.[25] Specifically, it has been shown to lower total cholesterol levels by as much as 30 percent, LDL cho-

---

What about Red Yeast Rice?

The red yeast (*Monascus purpureus*) fermented on rice is the source of monacolins, a group of compounds that are natural statins. In fact, the cholesterol-lowering prescription drug Mevacor (Merck) is the trade name for the compound lovastatin (also known as monacolin K), one of the key monacolins in red yeast rice extract.

The marketing of red yeast rice as a dietary supplement in the United States caused quite a controversy in 1997, since it contained a natural source of a prescription drug. The FDA and Merck eventually were able to prohibit the sale of red yeast rice extracts as a dietary supplement if the red yeast rice product contains significant amounts of lovastatin. And since a red yeast rice that did not contain lovastatin would probably not be effective, then a red yeast rice product that is effective at lowering cholesterol is probably in violation of federal law.

Here is my opinion. It just does not make sense to take red yeast rice. Lovastatin is now a generic drug and one of the least expensive statins. And if you are interested in taking an alternative to statins, there are definitely better choices than red yeast rice.

lesterol levels by 27 percent, and triglyceride levels by 34 percent within 4 to 12 weeks of use.

For best results, the recommended dosage is 400 mg of plant sterols plus 150 mg of Sytrinol twice daily. For larger individuals and for people with total cholesterol levels over 300 mg/dL, I generally recommend 1,200 of the plant sterols and 450 mg of Sytrinol daily.

The combination of plant sterols and Sytrinol is very safe for long-term use. The combination may enhance the performance of cholesterol-lowering drugs such as the statins, and can be used along with other natural cholesterol-lowering supplements such as niacin. Such combination products are available at your local health food store.

THE MOST IMPORTANT DIETARY SUPPLEMENT AGAINST CVD

Of all the nutritional products that can help prevent CVD, the most important, without question, is pharmaceutical-grade fish oil. The concept that eating fish may reduce the risk of heart disease began in the 1970s, when it was noted that among the Eskimos in arctic Greenland, where high consumption of marine animals was the normal diet, heart disease was very low. Subsequent studies in similar cultures where fish and seafood consumption was high showed the same sort of protection. For example, the inhabitants of the Japanese island of Okinawa, who eat primarily fish, were also observed to have a very low incidence of mortality from heart disease.

To assess the protective effects of fish against heart disease, researchers conducted large studies in which they tracked dietary intake of fish and other seafood over a long time. As the results of these studies became available in the mid-1980s and 1990s, they provided even stronger evidence that higher levels of fish consumption were associated with a lower risk of mortality from heart disease.

It is now estimated that individuals whose diets include a higher intake of fish oils, or who take fish oil supplements, can reduce their risk of heart disease or stroke by roughly 47 percent compared with individuals who do not eat fish or take fish oil supplements.[26, 27] In fact, the level of omega-3 fatty acids in the red blood cells (the omega-3 index) has been shown to be the most accurate predictor of the risk of heart disease and stroke.[28] It is a more sensitive indicator than other well-recognized markers, including cholesterol, LDL, HDL, CRP, and homocysteine. An omega-3 index of at least 8 percent is associated with the greatest protection against CVD.

Scientists now know that fish oils can also lower the risk of many cancers—particularly breast, prostate, colon, and lung cancer—and many other chronic diseases, including Alzheimer's disease, asthma, depression, diabetes, high blood pressure, macular degeneration, multiple sclerosis, and rheumatoid arthritis.[29]

FISH OR FISH OIL SUPPLEMENTS

Research assessing the amount of the important omega-3 fatty acids eicosapentaenoic acid (EPA) and docosahexaenoic acid (DHA) required to offer protection against heart disease (1,000 mg daily of EPA and DHA) suggests that the best way to achieve this goal is through supplementation. You simply cannot rely on fish to achieve this goal owing to the fact that mercury, PCBs, dioxins, and other contaminants are often found in fish. You need to limit your intake of fish to no more than two to three servings weekly. Follow these guidelines to reduce your chances of eating fish that is tainted with chemical toxins:

▸ Eat wild Pacific salmon as opposed to farm-raised salmon.

▸ Limit your intake of freshwater fish (particularly fish from inland lakes), as these are more likely to be contaminated with pesticides and carcinogens such as dioxin or PCBs. Lean ocean fish—cod, flounder, haddock etc.—are least likely to be contaminated.

▸ Eat smaller, young fish, as they have had less time to accumulate toxins in their fat.

▸ Check with the Department of Public Health before eating fish from nearby waters. It may be that local industries have polluted the water and caused unusually high levels of toxins in locally caught fish.

▶ If you are a sport fisherman and you fish the same area over and over, don't eat fish that you catch.

Keep in mind that nearly all fish contain trace amounts of methylmercury. The fish most likely to have the lowest level of methylmercury are salmon (usually undetectable levels), cod, cold-water tuna, farm-raised catfish, and herring. But certain seafood, particularly swordfish, mackerel, shark, and some other large predatory fish, may contain high levels of methylmercury. Fish absorb methylmercury from water and aquatic plants. Larger predatory fish also absorb mercury from their prey. Methylmercury binds tightly to the proteins in fish tissue, including muscle, and cooking does not reduce the mercury content significantly.

To sum up, high levels of contaminants such as mercury, PCBs, and dioxins in our environment and waters make eating certain fish on a regular basis extremely dangerous. That fact should not be taken to mean you should avoid fish entirely. Instead, make wise choices (in general, if you rely on wild Pacific salmon, you are very safe). Fish consumption is definitely a health-promoting dietary practice; however, it makes the most sense to rely on pharmaceutical-grade fish oils to achieve your daily intake of 1,000 mg combined for EPA and DHA.

Keep in mind that in order to represent itself truly as pharmaceutical-grade, a fish oil product must have the following characteristics:

▶ It must be manufactured in a certified Good Manufacturing Practices (GMP) facility approved for pharmaceutical products.

▶ It must be manufactured according to pharmaceutical standards, including quality control to ensure that the product is virtually free from lipid peroxides, heavy metals, environmental contaminants, and other harmful compounds.

▶ It must provide at least a 60 percent concentration of the most active long-chain omega-3 fatty acids (EPA and DHA).

Recommended Cholesterol and Triglyceride Levels (mg/dL)			
Factor	Desirable	Borderline	High-risk
Total cholesterol	200	200–239	≥240
LDL cholesterol	100–130	130–159	160
HDL cholesterol	≥60	35–59	<35
Triglycerides	150	150–199	≥200

HOW DO FISH OILS PREVENT CVD?

Contrary to popular opinion, fish oils have no significant effect on choles-terol levels or blood pressure. They do, however, have other effects that re-duce the risk of heart disease and strokes. For example, they have a powerful effect on lowering triglyceride levels. Triglycerides are another class of blood lipid (fats). In the past, the relationship between elevated triglyceride levels and CVD has been uncertain. Recently, however, a large body of accumu-lating evidence indicates that high triglyceride levels are an independent risk factor for CVD. This increased risk is the result of relationships between blood triglyceride levels and other risk factors, such as the presence of small dense low-density lipoprotein, insulin resistance, a tendency toward clot formation, and low-grade systemic inflammation. The effect of fish oils on lowering triglyceride levels can be astounding.[30] It is not uncommon for in-dividuals with extremely high triglyceride levels—500 to 600 mg/dL—to achieve levels below 150 mg/dL after four weeks of supplementing their diet with 1,000 to 3,000 mg daily of a combination of EPA and DHA from fish oils.

Fish oils also improve blood flow and reduce excessive stickiness of blood platelets. Once platelets adhere to each other, or aggregate, they re-lease potent compounds that dramatically promote the formation of ath-erosclerotic plaque. They can also form a clot, which can get stuck in small arteries and produce a heart attack or stroke. What determines the sticki-

Positive Relationships and Heart Health

Nutrition and lifestyle are important for a healthy heart, but perhaps even more important is developing and maintaining positive relationships. Good human relationships sustain us and nourish us—in body and soul. In fact, they are absolutely critical to heart health. Data from large, well-controlled studies have shown that loneliness, isolation, unfulfilling jobs, unfulfilling relationships, and a "broken heart" were as important risk factors for heart disease and premature death as smoking, high blood pressure, high blood cholesterol, obesity, and physical inactivity.[31]

Good scientific research, in this instance, is telling us something that most of us already know. We all need relationships and the love and acceptance that they should bring to us. In fact, the desire to be loved and appreciated is one of the main motivations of human behavior. Unfortunately, many of us do not always act in a manner that allows us to achieve something so vital to our existence.

ness of platelets is largely the type of fats in the diet. Whereas saturated fats and cholesterol increase platelet aggregation, omega-3 oils have the opposite effect.

FINAL COMMENTS

After reading this chapter, you may still be asking, What should I do? Here is what I would recommend:

- ▸ Do everything that you can to get your cholesterol levels into the ideal range without taking a statin drug first. Follow the dietary recommendations above. Try either the combination of plant sterols and Sytrinol or niacin. Either method typically produces reductions in total cholesterol level of 50 to 75 mg/dL in patients with initial total cholesterol levels above 250 mg/dL within the first two weeks. When the initial cholesterol level is above 300 mg/dL, I would recommend taking both the combination of Sytrinol and plant sterols and 1,500 to 2,000 mg of niacin.

▸ If your HDL level is less than 50 mg/dL, then definitely take 1,500 to 2,000 mg of niacin and get more exercise.

▸ If you are currently taking a statin drug or red yeast rice and your cholesterol levels are in the recommended range, I would recommend working with your doctor to start following the dietary recommendations and the combination of plant sterols and Sytrinol. After four to six weeks reduce the dosage of the statin by half. It is very important to recheck the cholesterol levels four weeks after reducing the statin dosage. If everything looks great, try eliminating the statin drug entirely and recheck in four weeks. You can always go back on the statin or add niacin if your cholesterol levels go up. If your cholesterol levels are not in the ideal range, even though you are on a statin, I would definitely recommend adding the niacin to your regimen. Continue to monitor your cholesterol levels with your doctor. In fact, if you continue to use a statin drug, taking niacin produces considerable benefits.

▸ If you must take a statin because it is medically indicated in your case, then you absolutely must supplement your diet with 100 to 200 mg of CoQ10 daily.

▸ Take a high-quality fish oil supplement at a dosage that will deliver 1,000 mg of EPA and DHA (combined) per day.

Also, keep in mind that regular physical exercise is extremely important in reducing the risk of heart disease and strokes. It accomplishes this goal by lowering cholesterol levels, improving the supply of blood and oxygen to the heart, increasing the functional capacity of the heart, reducing blood pressure, reducing obesity, and exerting a favorable effect on blood clotting.

8

DRUGS ARE LESS POWERFUL THAN OUR ATTITUDE

"The happiness of your life depends upon the quality of your thoughts: therefore, guard accordingly."
—Marcus Aurelius

DID YOU KNOW THAT one in four adults in the in the United States is likely to be on an antidepressant, an antianxiety drug, or some other psychoactive drug? To me, that is a staggering figure. It clearly indicates an epidemic, and a financial boon for drug makers. Drugs designed to make us feel better, relieve anxiety, or help us sleep are among the top sellers each year.

Since the introduction of Prozac in 1988, physicians have been prescribing the antidepressants known as selective serotonin reuptake inhibitors (SSRIs) as if they were M&Ms. These antidepressants—which also include Zoloft, Paxil, Luvox, Celexa, and Lexapro—are now among the world's most widely prescribed medications, with sales of about $20 billion per year in the United States alone.

In recent years, the side effects of these drugs, such as sexual dysfunction and suicidal behavior, have received a lot of attention. But before we get to the issue of side effects I want to focus on some very important questions. Can drugs really overcome a bad attitude and negative thinking? How effective are antidepressant drugs? Do they really improve the quality of life in the long run?

DO ANTIDEPRESSANT DRUGS REALLY WORK?

The allure of antidepressant drugs is the expectation that all your problems will magically go away when you take a little pill. The reality is that it is naive to think the matter is so simple. Belief in the magic of a pill, whether it is a placebo or an antidepressant, does seem to help relieve depression. But in all except the most severe cases there is really no difference in efficacy between the placebo and the drug. This conclusion is based on the success rate in double-blind studies comparing an antidepressant drug with a placebo. It does not matter which antidepressant you look at; whether it is Prozac or Celexa, its ability to benefit a patient with depression is only slightly better than that of a placebo, at best. This result is apparent even though the available research has probably been manipulated to produce the best possible outcome for the drug.

Remember that a placebo-controlled trial is designed to determine the true efficacy of a treatment. Placebo-controlled trials are thought to be especially critical in the investigation of drugs for psychiatric disorders because there really is no objective measurement for mental health or mental conditions—unlike conditions such as high cholesterol, high blood pressure, or diabetes. How a person "feels" is more difficult to measure than a laboratory value.

Of course, the placebo-controlled trial is also necessary in gaining the FDA's approval. The FDA requires at least two placebo-controlled trials with positive results but there is a loophole: there is no limit on the number of trial that fail to demonstrate the drug's superiority over a placebo. Perhaps the most striking example of this loophole was the approval of Prozac. As detailed in Dr. Peter Breggins's landmark book, *Talking Back to Prozac: What Doctors Aren't Telling You about Today's Most Controversial Drug*, Eli Lilly, the manufacturer of Prozac, initially sponsored 10 clinical trials. In six of these studies, the efficacy of this drug—which became a blockbuster—was no greater than that of a placebo. In the four positive studies submitted to the FDA, Prozac was tested in only 286 subjects. If you combine all the results of these initial 10 studies of Prozac, roughly 90 percent of the improvements reported by patients taking Prozac were also reported by the patients taking placebos.

In a very detailed analysis published in the British Medical Journal, "Efficacy of Antidepressants in Adults," two experts concluded "that selective serotonin reuptake inhibitors do not have a clinically meaningful advantage over placebo" and "have not been convincingly shown to affect the long term outcome of depression or suicide rates."[1] Furthermore, the researchers concluded that there should be a thorough reevaluation of current approaches to depression and further development of alternatives to drug treatment. These beliefs are not the rantings of extremists; they are thoughtful comments by recognized leaders, based on existing scientific evidence. These findings are actually quite consistent with many other detailed reviews by similar experts. Yet, as is the case with many other drugs, marketing by the drug companies overpowers the voice of medical reason.

The picture is even more disturbing if all the studies are examined. Manufacturers don't have to publish all their data in journals, but they do have to report every trial to the FDA. When researchers led by Dr. Irving Kirsch of the University of Connecticut petitioned the FDA under the Freedom of Information Act and received the full files on the six most widely prescribed antidepressants approved between 1987 and 1999 (Prozac, Zoloft, Paxil, Effexor, Serzone, and Celexa), they found that of the 47 trials conducted for these six drugs, only 20 showed any measurable advantage of the drugs over placebos—a much lower number than turns up in published research.[2] That is not surprising, because obviously the drug companies will suppress any negative studies that they paid for. All these studies used the same measure—the Hamilton Depression Rating Scale, which clinicians apply nearly universally to assess a patient's level of depression. If all the data are pooled, the average patient on drugs improved by about 10 points on the 52-point Hamilton scale, whereas patients on a placebo improved by a little more than eight points. A two-point difference is clinically meaningless, especially when the concerns over side effects are taken into consideration.

Depression Defined

Clinical depression is more than feeling depressed. The official definition given by the American Psychiatric Association in its *Diagnostic and Statistical Manual of Mental Disorders (DSM-VIII)*, is based on eight primary criteria:

1. Poor appetite with weight loss, or increased appetite with weight gain
2. Insomnia or hypersomnia (wanting to sleep all the time)
3. Physical hyperactivity or inactivity
4. Loss of interest or pleasure in usual activities, or decrease in sexual drive
5. Loss of energy and feelings of fatigue
6. Feelings of worthlessness, self-reproach, or inappropriate guilt
7. Diminished ability to think or concentrate
8. Recurrent thoughts of death or suicide

The presence of five of these eight symptoms definitely indicates clinical depression; an individual with four symptoms is probably depressed. According to *DSM-VIII*, the condition must be present for at least one month to be called depression. Clinical depression is also referred to as major depression or unipolar depression.

HOW DID PROZAC AND OTHER SSRIS GET TO BE SUCH BIG BUSINESS?

Hailed as a medical miracle by many and deplored as a dangerous psychoactive drug by others, Prozac is perhaps the most controversial drug ever marketed. Developed by Eli Lilly and Company, Prozac was launched in the United States in 1987. It quickly became the most widely prescribed (and most profitable antidepressant drug. Though antidepressant drugs like Prozac are no more effective than a placebo, they are certainly more expensive.

The monthly cost of Prozac and other SSRIs can range between $50 and $200, depending on the dosage.

Why did Prozac become so popular? The media have played a major role by publishing articles describing Prozac as a breakthrough in the treatment of depression. The public, hungry for information about this miraculous "happy pill," kept the psychiatrist Peter Kramer's pro-Prozac book, *Listening to Prozac*, on the *New York Times* best-seller list for nearly four months in 1987. Dr. Kramer advocated Prozac for "cosmetic psychopharmacology" and in helping a normal person develop a more "socially rewarding personality." According to him, "Prozac seems to fire confidence to the habitually timid, to make the sensitive brash, to lend the introvert the social skills of a salesman." Of course, Dr. Kramer also points out that not all patients respond this way.

Another reason for the widespread popularity off SSRIs in recent years is that Prozac and other antidepressant drugs fit nicely into the dominant theoretical model of depression—the "biogenic amine" hypothesis. This model focuses more on biochemical factors in the brain than on psychological factors. Perhaps the main reason this model is so popular is that it is a better fit with drug therapy. According to the biogenic amine hypothesis, depression is caused by biochemical imbalances of amino acids, which form neurotransmitters known as monoamines. Monoamines include serotonin, melatonin, gamma-aminobutyric acid (GABA), dopamine, and norepinephrine. Environmental, nutritional, psychological, and genetic factors can all lead to an imbalance in the monoamines that might result in depression. Monoamine neurotransmitters are released by brain cells to carry a chemical message from one nerve cell to another by binding to receptor sites on neighboring brain cells. Different antidepressant drugs act by increasing different monoamines in the brain either through blocking the reuptake, blocking the breakdown, or enhancing the effect of a specific monoamine.

It is interesting to note that the monoamines are manufactured from dietary amino acids—the building-block molecules of proteins. For example, the amino acid tryptophan serves as the precursor to serotonin and melatonin; and phenylalanine and tyrosine are precursors to dopamine, epinephrine, and norepinephrine. These amino acids have proved to be effective natural antidepressants and are discussed in Chapter 9.

HOW DO SSRIS WORK?

The SSRIs are thought to work by specifically inhibiting the reuptake of serotonin at the nerve endings in the brain. As a result, more serotonin is likely to bind to receptor sites on brain cells and transmit the serotonin signal. Serotonin is a very important neurotransmitter. It is the brain's own natural antidepressant and tranquilizer. A decrease in serotonin function is thought to be a major cause of depression, anxiety, and insomnia.

Not only serotonin is important in controlling your moods and behavior; it also acts as a kind of chemical traffic cop to regulate the activity of many other neurotransmitters. The level of serotonin present in your brain can have a tremendous impact on how you think, feel, and behave.

Effects of Different Levels of Serotonin

Optimal Level of Serotonin	Low Level of Serotonin
Hopeful, optimistic	Depressed
Calm	Anxious
"Good-natured"	Irritable
Patient	Impatient
Reflective and thoughtful	Impulsive
Loving and caring	Abusive
Able to concentrate	Short attention span
Creative, focused	Blocked, scattered
Able to think things through	"Flies off the handle"
Responsive	Reactive

| Does not overeat carbohydrates | Craves sweets and high-carbohydrate foods |
| Sleeps well with good recall of dreams | Insomnia and poor recall of dreams |

The lower your level of serotonin, the more severe and widespread the potential impact on your brain and body. For example, low levels of serotonin can cause an overwhelming craving for sugar. Research has shown that many people with bulimia, an eating disorder characterized by uncontrollable eating binges, have insufficient supplies of serotonin.

Conditions Associated with Low Serotonin Levels

- Aggression
- Alcoholism
- Anxiety
- Attention deficit disorder
- Bulimia
- Carbohydrate cravings
- Chronic pain disorders (such as fibromyalgia)
- Depression
- Epilepsy
- Headaches (migraines, tension headaches, chronic headaches)
- Hyperactivity
- Insomnia
- Myoclonus (muscle twitching)
- Obesity

- ▶ Obsessive-compulsive disorder

- ▶ Panic disorders

- ▶ Premenstrual syndrome

- ▶ Schizophrenia

- ▶ Seasonal affective disorder ("winter depression")

- ▶ Suicidal thoughts and behavior

The problems arising from serotonin deficiency syndrome may vary from person to person. For example, in some people, low levels of serotonin may cause depression; in others, the same level of serotonin might produce regular disabling headaches or a voracious appetite for sweets and carbohydrates.

These variations in the effects of serotonin reflect human biochemical individuality. Although we all have the same basic electrochemical wiring system in our brains, there are major differences in how we respond, in terms of mood and behavior, to the signals sent along that system.

You might be wondering: if serotonin is so important, why can't I just increase my level by taking a pill or having an injection? The simple answer is that serotonin cannot be "imported" to the brain from outside. It can only be manufactured within the brain. We can, however, improve the manufacture of serotonin within the brain.

SIDE EFFECTS OF PROZAC AND OTHER ANTIDEPRESSANT DRUGS

Antidepressant drugs are only marginally successful in alleviating depression in many cases, and they do have many side effects. Approximately 20 percent of patients experience nausea; 20 percent headaches; 15 percent anxiety and nervousness; 14 percent insomnia; 12 percent drowsiness; 12 percent diarrhea; 9.5 percent dry mouth; 9 percent loss of appetite; 8 percent sweating and tremor; and 3 percent rash. The SSRIs also definitely inhibit sexual function. In studies where sexual side effects were thoroughly

Boosting Serotonin Levels Naturally

You may not need drugs to boost your serotonin levels; here are some good natural approaches:

▸ Psychological therapy has been shown to be as effective as antidepressant drugs in treating moderate depression.[3]

▸ It is important to rule out the simple organic factors that are known to contribute to low serotonin levels, i.e., nutrient deficiency or excess, drugs (prescription, illicit, alcohol, caffeine, nicotine, etc.), hypoglycemia, hormonal derangement, allergy, and environmental factors.

▸ Depression is often a first or early manifestation of low thyroid function.[4] Thyroid hormone appears to be necessary in the conversion of tryptophan to serotonin.

▸ Elimination of sugar and caffeine has been shown to produce significant benefits in clinical trials in patients with depression.[5] This effect is due to improving the conversion of tryptophan to serotonin as well as other mechanisms.

▸ Increased participation in exercise, sports, and physical activities is strongly associated with decreased symptoms of anxiety, depression, and malaise, indicating an association with higher serotonin levels.[6]

▸ 5-Hydroxytryptophan (5-HTP) is the direct precursor to serotonin that is able to cross the blood-brain barrier and raise brain serotonin levels. As a result, supplementing the diet with 5-HTP has been shown to produce significant benefits in conditions linked to low serotonin, including depression, weight loss, headaches, and fibromyalgia.[7] The starting dosage should be 50 milligrams (mg) three times per day. If the response is inadequate after two weeks, the dosage can be increased to 100 mg three times per day. Be sure to use 5-HTP in enteric-coated capsules or tablets (pills prepared so that they will not dissolve in the stomach); they significantly reduce the likelihood of nausea.

▸ Consider taking St. John's-wort according to the guidelines given on page 168.

evaluated, 43 percent of men and women taking SSRIs reported loss of libido or diminished sexual response.

The SSRIs also can produce "akathisia," a drug-induced state of agitation. In some people, this may lead to violent, destructive outbursts. By 1990, the violent and suicidal reactions experienced by some patients taking Prozac became so common and so well publicized that several citizens' groups were formed to create awareness of these dangers of the drug, most notably the Citizens' Commission on Human Rights.

Because of the negative publicity, the FDA convened a special committee to examine the growing concerns about Prozac. However, independent reviews of the proceedings of this committee clearly show a bias toward supporting the presentations from Eli Lilly. In fact, when Dr. Martin Teicher, a researcher at Harvard, began to give evidence of a possible link between Prozac and violent, suicidal thoughts, the panel at the FDA hearing refused to allow him to present his slides. Of course, the fact that nine of the 10 members of the panel had a conflict of interest—they had received money from the drug companies being represented—may have influenced their decision. For example, the psychiatrist David Dunner had direct financial compensation of more than $500,000 from four manufacturers of antidepressants and more than $4 million worth of research grants from manufacturers of antidepressants in an eight-year period. Remarkably, Dr. Dunner even had $200,000 worth of grants "pending" from Eli Lilly, Prozac's manufacturer, when the hearing took place.

Even though this FDA committee rejected the association between Prozac and suicide in 1990, the issue was never completely settled. It remains a very controversial association. Another reason why the FDA committee may have rejected the association was the clever way the drug companies hid it. Every antidepressant licensed by the FDA since 1987 showed an excess of suicides compared with a placebo, but the manufacturers included all suicides that occurred after the subjects were enrolled in the study, but before they were assigned to a treatment group or to the placebo group.[8]

Some studies have not shown an association between SSRIs and suicide, but these studies are offset by other studies and numerous case reports suggesting a very strong link. Although results vary, there is a very consistent trend. Compared with a placebo, all SSRIs seem to at least double the risk of suicidal thinking, from 1–2 percent to 2–4 percent, in both children and adults, and the real impact may be much greater.[9]

In October 2004, after much hesitation, and under pressure from parents and Congress, the FDA finally issued a "Black Box Warning" for physicians and pharmacists—its strongest available measure short of withdrawing a drug from the market. The warning is placed on package inserts for all antidepressants in common use. It mentions the risk of suicidal thoughts, hostility, and agitation in both children and adults, specifically citing statistical analyses of clinical trials. The FDA has also issued a public advisory to parents, physicians, and pharmacists.

One of the interesting findings from this focus on children and SSRIs was that children and adolescents received about a third of all antidepressant prescriptions in the United States. This is shocking, given that the effects of long-term use of these drugs on still developing brains is unknown. Fortunately, the warnings and regulations quickly and definitely influenced the number of antidepressant prescriptions for children.[10] And, although there have been some reports in the medical literature and the popular media suggesting an increase in childhood suicides, according to current available evidence that is not the case. Preliminary statistics from the National Center for Health Statistics for 2005 show that the number of suicides actually declined for children, adolescents, and young adults despite the big drop in the number of prescriptions being written.

SSRIS AND WEIGHT GAIN

Another side effect of SSRIs that was once highly controversial is weight gain. I had many patients come to see me seeking an alternative to SSRIs because they felt these drugs were responsible for their rapid, dramatic weight gain. At the time, their medical doctors were telling them there was no association between these drugs and weight gain, but I told them the exact opposite. Too many patients had told me the same thing for it to be a coincidence. Only recently has weight gain from SSRIs been firmly accepted in many medical circles, and it is still not listed as a side effect in information regarding prescriptions. Statistics show that once weight gain begins while a patient is taking these medications, it usually does not stop. Not uncommonly, people report that they have gained 40 to 60 pounds in a short time.

These drugs induce weight gain because they alter an area of the brain that regulates both serotonin levels and the utilization of glucose.[11] The human brain is usually only 2 percent of overall body mass, but it is so metabolically active that it uses up to 50 percent of the glucose in the body for energy. Evidently the SSRIs disrupt the utilization of glucose in the brain, and the brain then senses that it is low in glucose. This situation sets in motion very powerful signals to eat. Typically, if a person has had cravings for sugar or other foods they will be dramatically intensified by the drug. Other changes produced by the drug lead to insulin resistance, setting the stage for inevitable weight gain, and perhaps even type 2 diabetes. Studies have shown that individuals predisposed to diabetes are two to three times more likely to become diabetic if they use an antidepressant medication.[12]

WHATEVER HAPPENED TO ST. JOHN'S-WORT?

In the late 1990s the brightest star in herbal medicine was without question St. John's-wort extract. In fact, in Germany in 1996 it was estimated that physicians prescribed St. John's-wort extract eight times more frequently than Prozac for the treatment of depression. In the United States, on June 27, 1997, the television news show 20/20 included a segment called "Nature's Rx: Using Herb St. John's-Wort to Treat Depression." This brought considerable attention not only to St. John's-wort extract (SJWE) but to herbal medicine in general. The increased popularity of this safe, effective natural product certainly did not go unnoticed by drug manufacturing executives.

In April 2001, however, there was a blaring headline on the cover of *Time* magazine: "St. John's-What?" The accompanying article reported a study which had found that St. John's-Wort didn't work any better than a placebo.[13] However, this study involved 200 patients with severe depression of at least two years' duration—not the typical mild to moderate depression for which other studies had clearly demonstrated significant benefits from SJWE. Many experts felt that in the study reported by *Time*, the researchers seemed to have stacked the deck against SJWE. Interestingly, the funding of the study came from a giant drug company, Pfizer, the maker of Zoloft—the number one antidepressant drug at the time. There was much criticism of this study, for good reason. It was out of line with other studies then and since (more than 30 double-blind studies) examining mild to moderate depression. Also, it is important to repeat that the subjects selected for the Pfizer study had severe depression lasting at least two years and were not likely to respond to any treatment. Even so, significantly more patients had a remission of illness with SJWE than with a placebo; however, the overall success rates for both were very low (14.3 percent for SJWE; 5 percent for the placebo).

Since this study comparing SJWE with Zoloft for severe depression, there have been several double-blind studies comparing SJWE with standard SSRIs, including Zoloft, for mild to moderate depression. These studies have shown that SJWE is more effective and has fewer side effects.[14, 15] The message from all this research is that for severe cases of depression, SJWE may not be strong enough. These patients may be better off initially using conventional antidepressant drugs to prevent harm to themselves or others until they begin to respond to cognitive therapy (see below).

POOR QUALITY ALSO LED TO A DECLINE IN THE POPULARITY OF SJWE

Another reason why the reputation of SJWE became somewhat tarnished is that many people did not experience the expected results. In many cases unrealistic expectations may have led to the perception that SJWE was disappointing. No pill can dramatically change one's circumstances in life, yet many people seemed to expect that if they simply took SJWE their lives would magically improve. Although SJWE and other antidepressant agents can help improve one's outlook and perspective, expecting much more is a bit unrealistic.

Another cause of the downturn in popularity, in my opinion, was the poor quality of some products on the market. I have stressed relentlessly for

25 years that the effectiveness of any herbal product (or any drug, for that matter) is based on delivering an effective dosage of active compounds. If you want to see the same results noted in the numerous clinical trials with SJWE, it is absolutely essential that you use the same quality of extract used in the studies. The extracts used in the studies were typically standardized to contain 0.3 percent hypericin and 3 to 5 percent hyperforin. Although hypericin and hyperforin are important components, this extract is composed of a wide range of compounds constituting the remaining 95 percent. Manufacturers of high-quality SJWE apply analytical techniques to identify not only the hypericin and hyperforin, but also several other crucial components. The point is that although the extracts are standardized for the marker compounds, ensuring appropriate levels of these other constituents is also vitally important.

Various independent analyses, by *Consumer Reports*, *Orange County Register*, and other demonstrated that the market was full of poor-quality SJWE. And, even if a product had the proper level of the marker compounds hypericin and hyperforin, there was no real guarantee that it was the same quality as the clinically proven extracts. The quality of SJWE varies tremendously even though the labels of two different SJWEs may state the same level of the marker compounds. Typically, higher-quality clinically tested SJWE is three to four times more expensive than a raw material.

The point here is that many people may not have experienced the benefits that SJWE had to offer because they were not using an effective product. As there is no real way for consumers to know all the intricate details of what goes into SJWE, it is imperative that they rely on respected health food store brands.

SJWE: DOSAGE AND SIDE EFFECTS

The dosage for the SJWE standardized to contain 0.3 percent hypericin and 3 to 5 percent hyperforin is typically 900 mg per day for mild depression and 1,800 mg per day for moderate to severe depression. Initially the dosage was spread out during the day, but recent studies indicate that a single daily dose is preferable.

With regard to side effects, according to a large body of clinical data SJWE is remarkably safe, with no significant side effects reported in the numerous double-blind studies. In contrast, side effects such as weight gain, sedation, gastrointestinal disturbances, and sexual dysfunction are often experienced by patients treated with antidepressant drugs.

The frequency and severity of side effects with SJWE are clinically insignificant, especially when compared with the well-known side effects of tricyclics and other antidepressants. There have been no deaths due to toxicity of SJWE—a stark contrast with the 31 deaths per 1 million prescriptions for synthetic antidepressants.

One potential side effect that continues to get a lot of attention is photosensitivity (reactions to sunlight). However, the amount of hypericin ingested at recommended levels is about 20 to 50 times below the level required to produce phototoxicity.

Potential drug interactions with SJWE are a reality. Because SJWE can increase the activity of a drug detoxifying enzyme in the liver, it has been found to decrease the plasma concentrations of a long list of drugs. As a general rule, if you are taking any prescription medication, including birth control pills, do not take SJWE without the approval of your physician.

DISCONTINUING SSRIS

After reading all this information, if you are taking an SSRI, you may want to stop. This is a good goal, but I don't want to imply that I think the best treatment for depression is no treatment. Especially in severe depression, an SSRI may be an appropriate therapy. I also must tell you that discontinuing an SSRI has to be done gradually. Stopping too quickly is associated with symptoms such as dizziness, uncoordination, fatigue, tingling, burning, blurred vision, insomnia, and vivid dreams. Less often, there may be nausea or diarrhea, flu-like symptoms, irritability, anxiety, and crying spells. The drug industry and the medical profession prefer to use the term "discontinuation syndrome" to describe these symptoms, but my response is, Let's get real. These symptoms are classic withdrawal reactions that are associated with drug addictions.

To help support patients as they go off SSRIs, I typically will recommend either 5-HTP or SJWE. I have used these natural products successfully and without incident for patients taking Prozac, Zoloft, Paxil, Effexor, and various other antidepressant drugs. The real concern in mixing antidepressant drugs with SJWE or 5-HTP is producing the "serotonin syndrome"—a condition characterized by confusion, fever, shivering, sweating, diarrhea, and muscle spasms. Although it is theoretically possible that combining SJWE or 5-HTP with standard antidepressant drugs could produce this syndrome, to my knowledge no one has experienced the syndrome in that situation. Nonetheless, my recommendation is that if you are using SJWE or 5-HTP in combination with standard antidepressant drugs, you should be closely monitored by your doctor for any reactions suggestive of serotonin syndrome. If these symptoms appear, elimination of one of the therapies is indicated.

In mild cases of depression, I would recommend using either 5-HTP (50 mg per day) or SJWE extract (900 mg daily) while reducing the drug to half the daily dosage for two to four weeks. After this time, totally eliminate the drug. For more severe cases, keep the dosage of the antidepressant as it is and add SJWE. Then, evaluate at the end of one month and begin tapering off the drug if sufficient mood-elevating effects have been noted. If additional support is necessary, I usually add 5-HTP at a dosage of 50 mg three times daily.

A DIFFERENT VIEW OF DEPRESSION

Modern psychiatry focuses on correcting the chemical changes in the neurotransmitters of the brain that produce depression through drug therapy, rather than identifying and eliminating the psychological factors that are responsible for producing imbalances in serotonin, dopamine, GABA, and other neurotransmitters. There are physiological reasons for these imbalances, but in most cases the real secret to eliminating depression is utilizing techniques and therapies that help the depressed individual learn life skills and develop a more optimistic outlook.

Of all of the different models of human depression, the one that I feel has the most merit is the learned helplessness model developed by Martin Seligman, Ph.D. I believe that Dr. Seligman's contributions to the understanding of human behavior are on par with Albert Einstein's contributions to physics and Linus Pauling's contributions to biochemistry. If you are interested in learning more about this eminent scientist, I encourage you to read his classic book *Learned Optimism* (Knopf, 1991).

One of Dr. Seligman's major contributions to psychology was the development of the "learned helplessness model of depression," as an animal model is known. During the 1960s, Dr. Seligman discovered that animals could be trained to be helpless. What significance do these experiments have for depression? Seligman's learned helplessness model became an effective way to test antidepressant drugs. Basically, when animals that had learned to be helpless were given antidepressant drugs, they would unlearn helplessness and start exerting control over their environment. Scientists discovered that when animals learned to be helpless, this learning resulted in alteration of brain monoamine content: e.g., it lowered brain serotonin levels. The drugs would restore proper monoamine balance and alter the animal's behavior. Researchers also found that when animals with learned helplessness were taught how to gain control over their environment, brain chemistry also normalized.

The alteration in brain monoamine content in the animals with learned helplessness mirrors the altered monoamine content in human depression. What all the research indicates is that learned helplessness in animals and depression in humans can be improved either by antidepressant drugs or through retraining.

Most physicians quickly look to drugs to alter brain chemistry, but helping patients gain greater control over their lives will actually produce even greater biochemical changes. One of the most powerful techniques for producing the necessary biochemical changes in the brain of depressed individuals is teaching them to be more optimistic.

Outside the laboratory setting, Dr. Seligman discovered that the factor determining how people would react to an uncontrollable event, either "bad" or "good," was their explanatory style—the way they explained events. Optimistic people were immune to becoming helpless and depressed. However, individuals who were pessimistic were extremely likely to become depressed when something went wrong in their lives. Dr. Seligman and other researchers also found a direct correlation between an individual's level of optimism and the likelihood of developing not only clinical depression but other illnesses as well. In one of the longer studies, patients were followed for a total of 35 years. Optimists rarely became depressed, but pessimists were extremely likely to develop depression and other psychological disturbances.

To determine whether you are an optimist or a pessimist, I encourage you to fill out Seligman's questionnaire in Appendix A on pages 263–269. If you are a pessimist you are likely to be depressed, and if you are depressed you are likely to be a pessimist.

COGNITIVE THERAPY

A number of psychological therapies can be quite useful in helping to eliminate depression. The therapy that I feel has the most merit and support is cognitive therapy. In fact, cognitive therapy has been shown to be superior to antidepressant drugs in treating mild to moderate depression.[3] In addition, whereas there is a high rate of recurrence of depression when drugs are used, the relapse rate with cognitive therapy is much lower. People taking drugs for depression tend to have to stay on them for the rest of their lives. That is not the case with cognitive therapy, because the patient is taught new skills to deal with depression.

Psychologists and other mental health specialists trained in cognitive therapy seek to change the way the depressed person consciously thinks about failure, defeat, loss, and helplessness. Cognitive therapists apply five basic tactics.

First, they help patients recognize the negative automatic thoughts that flit through consciousness at the times when the patients feel worst. Second, they dispute the negative thoughts by focusing on contrary evidence. Third, they teach the patient a different explanation, to dispel the negative automatic thoughts. Fourth, they help the patients to better control thoughts by learning how to avoid rumination (the constant churning of a thought in the mind). Fifth; they help patients to question negative thoughts and beliefs and to replace these with empowering positive thoughts and beliefs.

Cognitive therapy does not involve the long-drawn-out process of psychoanalysis. It is a solution-oriented psychotherapy designed to help the patient learn skills that will improve the quality of his or her life. If your thought processes are in need of rewiring, please consult a mental health specialist who practices cognitive therapy.

RULING OUT AN ORGANIC CAUSE

In Chapter 3, I noted that one failure of conventional medicine is an inability to identify and eliminate obstacles to a cure. In that light, depression can be due to an underlying organic or physiological cause. It is essential to rule out or eliminate easily reversible organic causes of depression before taking any antidepressant drug. In particular, depression is often a side effect of a medical condition or of prescription drugs. Common drugs associated with depression include corticosteroids, beta-blockers, and other antihypertensive medications. In addition, substances not often considered drugs such as oral contraceptives, alcohol, caffeine, and cigarettes can also cause depression. All these drugs disrupt the normal balance between brain neurotransmitters. If you are taking any medication, consult the *Physician's Desk Reference*, the Internet, or your pharmacist about the possibility that the drug might cause depression as a side effect. For most health conditions, there are natural medicines that may produce better results than drugs, without side effects.

Organic and Physiological Causes of Depression

Preexisting Physical Conditions

Diabetes	Rheumatoid arthritis
Heart disease	Chronic inflammation
Lung disease	Chronic pain

Cancer	Multiple sclerosis
Liver disease	

Drugs, Prescription

Antihypertensives	Antihistamines
Anti-inflammatory agents	Corticosteroids
Birth control pills	Tranquilizers and sedatives

Other Causes

Premenstrual syndrome	Hypothyroidism
Stress or low adrenal function	Hypoglycemia
Heavy metals	Nutritional deficiencies
Food allergies	Sleep disturbances

DON'T UNDERESTIMATE THE
IMPORTANCE OF SLEEP

Adequate sleep is absolutely necessary for long-term health and regeneration. Many physiologic processes occur during sleep, so without sufficient sleep our body and mind do not get recharged. Poor quality of sleep is a huge issue in America; it is estimated that more than 60 percent of adults in the United States have sleep problems a few nights a week or more. In addition, more than 40 percent of adults experience daytime sleepiness severe enough to interfere with their daily activities at least a few days each month—and 20 percent report problematic sleepiness a few days a week or more. At least 40 million Americans suffer from sleep disorders, yet more than 60 percent of adults have never been asked about the quality of their sleep by a physician and fewer than 20 percent have ever initiated a discussion.

The importance of sleep to our moods is obvious, but often overlooked. I know that for me it is more challenging to be positive, joyful, and passionate if I do not get a good night's sleep. I am sure you feel the same way. My feeling is that the quality of our sleep is directly proportional to the quality of our mood and our life. Having children made me realize just how important sleep is to moods. I noticed its effect not only in my life, but also in my kids' lives. My son, Zachary, loved to sleep and was always in a good mood with a big smile on his face. My oldest daughter, Lexi, did not sleep as well. Her mood would be clearly affected by how well she had slept. Now that she is a teenager, I see that correlation even more. When she does not get enough sleep, it is easy for her to get a bit off balance, get stressed out, and overreact. Trust me: high-quality sleep is very, very important to all of us, and especially to teenagers. Examine the role of sleep in your own life. Here are seven tips for improving the quality of sleep.

Seven Tips for a Good Night's Sleep

1. Make your bedroom primarily a place for sleeping. It is not a good idea to use your bed for paying bills, doing work, etc. Help your body recognize that this is a place for rest or intimacy. Make sure your room is well ventilated and the temperature is consistent. And try to keep it quiet. You could use a fan or a white-noise machine to help block outside noises.

2. Incorporate bedtime rituals. Listening to soft music or sipping a cup of herbal tea cues your body that it's time to slow down and begin to prepare for sleep. Try to go to bed and wake up at the same time every day, even on weekends. Keeping a regular schedule will help your body expect sleep at the same time each day. Don't oversleep to make up for a poor night's sleep—doing that for even a couple of days can reset your body clock and make it hard for you to get to sleep at night.

3. Relax for a while before going to bed. Spending quiet time can make falling asleep easier. This may include meditation, relaxation, breathing exercises, or taking a warm bath. Try listening to recorded relaxation or guided imagery programs.

4. Get out of bed if you are unable to sleep. Don't lie in bed awake. Go into another room and do something relaxing until you feel sleepy. Worrying about falling asleep actually keeps many people awake.

5. Don't do anything stimulating. Don't read anything job-related or watch a stimulating television program (commercials and news shows tend to be stimulating). Don't expose yourself to bright light. The light gives cues to your brain that it is time to wake up.

6. Perform progressive relaxation. This technique is based on a very simple procedure of comparing tension with relaxation. Begin with contracting the muscles of the face and neck, hold the contraction for a period of at least one to two seconds, and then relax the muscles. Next the upper arms and chest are contracted and then relaxed, followed by the lower arms and hands. Repeat the process progressively down the body: i.e., the abdomen, the buttocks, the thighs, the calves, and the feet. Then work your way back up to your head. Repeat two or three times. This technique is often used in the treatment of anxiety and insomnia.

7. Use a natural product to improve the quality of sleep. A number of natural products can help to improve sleep. The specific product that I recommend is Tranquil Sleep from Natural Factors: it provides a combination of melatonin, 5-HTP, and L-theanine in a great-tasting chewable tablet. Melatonin is an important hormone secreted by the pineal gland, a small gland in the center of the brain. If a person's melatonin levels are low, melatonin at bedtime can produce a gentle sedative effect. A dosage of 3 mg at bedtime is more than enough. The amino acids 5-HTP and L-theanine (a relaxing compound from green tea) have been shown to decrease the time required to get to sleep and to decrease the number of nighttime awakenings, and they really seem to work well with melatonin. The recommended dosage at bedtime is 30 to 60 mg for 5-HTP and 200 to 400 mg for L-theanine. Although I recommend the Tranquil Sleep formula for adults, I have found that kids really respond well to L-theanine alone.

FINAL COMMENTS

One of the first books that I read concerning "alternative medicine" was Dr. Kenneth Pelletier's *Mind as Healer, Mind as Slayer*, written in 1977 and revised in 1992. This book is a classic that should be on every doctor's bookshelf, along with Dr. Pelletier's *Sound Mind, Sound Body—A New Model for Lifelong Health.*

Although *Sound Mind, Sound Body* was written for the public, I believe it should be required reading for any health care practitioner. Dr. Pelletier has done a masterful job of presenting the importance of a positive, purposeful life orientation to lifelong good health. Among his findings:

▶ There is a healthy way of being ill, which can help a person manage chronic disease such as rheumatoid arthritis and heart disease.

▶ People who overcome serious illness or physical trauma in childhood are often actually strengthened—not debilitated—by the experience.

▶ Altruistic work is closely related to the ability to overcome life-threatening crises and disease.

▶ Positive relationships are critical to achieving and maintaining good health.

Dr. Pelletier is now a clinical professor of medicine at the University of Arizona School of Medicine; he was formerly at the Stanford University School of Medicine. In *Sound Mind, Sound Body*, he draws from the results of recent research findings as well as his own five-year Rockefeller-funded study of 51 prominent men and women who have made major contributions to the world beyond their own personal successes.

Dr. Pelletier's work is reminiscent of Abraham Maslow, the American psychologist who in 1943 brought us the concept of self-actualization—a process of ongoing actualization of our potentials, capacities, and talents. Maslow was really the first psychologist to study healthy people. He strongly believed that the study of healthy people would create a firm foundation for the theories and values of a new psychotherapy. His work and theories were the result of intense research on psychologically healthy people during a period of more than 30 years. Maslow discovered that healthy individuals strive and are actually driven to be self-actualized. He found that self-actualized people had the following traits which are certainly worth striving for in our lives:

- They embrace the facts and realities of the world (including themselves) rather than denying or avoiding them.

- They are spontaneous in their ideas and actions.

- They are creative.

- They are interested in solving problems; these often include the problems of others. Solving these problems is often a key focus in their lives.

- They feel close to other people, and generally appreciate life.

- They have a system of morality that is fully internalized and independent of external authority.

- They have discernment and are able to view all things in an objective manner.

9

DRUGS CANNOT OVERCOME A POOR DIET OR AN UNHEALTHY LIFESTYLE

"Let your food be your medicine and let your medicine be your food."

—Hippocrates

THERE IS AN EVER-GROWING appreciation of the role of diet in determining our level of health. It is now well established that certain dietary practices cause, and others prevent, a wide range of diseases. In addition, more and more research indicates certain diets and foods offer immediate therapeutic benefits. Yet despite these advances, rarely are patients with diet-related diseases given the dietary information that could lead them to better health. Instead, people with diabetes, high blood pressure, and many other diet-related diseases are immediately placed on drug regimens. And what the drug companies won't tell you and your doctor doesn't know about these drug regimens is that they ultimately cripple our body processes and shorten our lives. As startling as that statement may seem, it is nonetheless irrefutable.

Natural medicine may not provide all the answers for every person with type 2 diabetes or high blood pressure, but there is no way around the fact that no drug provides all the benefits a person can achieve through diet, lifestyle, and key natural medicines. Although drugs may be necessary in some cases, they simply cannot replace the many advantages produced by diet and lifestyle.

METABOLIC SYNDROME—
AN AMERICAN EPIDEMIC

It is estimated that about 60 million adults in the United States meet the criteria for metabolic syndrome. This cluster of signs and symptoms includes:

▸ Central obesity (excessive fat tissue in and around the abdomen) as demonstrated by a greater waist-to-hip ratio.

▸ Low levels of HDL cholesterol—less than 40 milligrams per deciliter (mg/dL) in men and less than 50 mg/dL in women.

▸ Fasting blood triglycerides of 150 mg/dL or more.

▸ Elevated blood pressure (130/85 mm Hg or higher).

▸ Insulin resistance (the body can't properly use insulin or blood glucose), as demonstrated by the presence of prediabetes (glucose levels between 101 and 125 mg/dL)

▸ Elevated uric acid levels (above 8.3 mg/dL).

Originally referred to as "syndrome X" by the endocrinologist Gerald Reaven, M.D., of Stanford University, metabolic syndrome is a serious health issue because people who have it are at increased risk of coronary artery disease, other diseases related to plaque buildup in artery walls (e.g., stroke and peripheral vascular disease), and type 2 diabetes. The presence of four or more of the above criteria is associated with a 2.5 times greater risk of a heart attack or stroke, and a nearly 25 times greater risk of diabetes.

Metabolic syndrome, prediabetes, hypoglycemia, increased insulin secretion, and even type 2 diabetes can be viewed as different facets of the same disease having the same underlying dietary, lifestyle, and genetic causes. The human body was simply not designed to handle the amount of

---

Fast-Food and Insulin Resistance

Given the relationship between obesity and the incidence of type 2 diabetes, researchers sought to assess the association between fast food, weight gain, and insulin resistance in a study called Coronary Artery Risk Development in Young Adults (CARDIA). The results showed that those participants who frequented fast-food restaurants more than two times per week at the start of the study and at the 15-year follow-up put on an extra 10 pounds and had an approximately 200 percent greater increase in insulin resistance than participants who ate at fast-food restaurants less than once a week at baseline and follow-up. These findings demonstrate that fast-food is strongly linked to weight gain and insulin resistance.[1]

---

refined sugar, white flour, salt, saturated fats, and other harmful food compounds that many people in the United States and other western countries consume, especially when such a diet is combined with a sedentary lifestyle. The result is that a metabolic syndrome emerges—elevated insulin levels, obesity, elevated blood cholesterol and triglycerides, and high blood pressure. "Metabolic syndrome" is the label modern medicine has chosen to ascribe to a condition caused by poor dietary and lifestyle choices. It seems rather silly for medical researchers to be spending millions of dollars on the development of drugs (presumed to be "magic bullets") to address these problems, when they could be prevented at far less cost, and far more effectively, by teaching people how to choose a healthier diet and lifestyle. It is highly unlikely that there will ever be a drug to replace the important dietary and lifestyle factors on which the human body lives and thrives.

METABOLIC SYNDROME IS A GOLD MINE FOR THE DRUG INDUSTRY

Patients with metabolic syndrome are a virtual gold mine for the drug industry. Typically, these patients are on very extensive (and expensive) drug regimens to try to address the many facets of this syndrome. Here is a typical list of drugs prescribed for patients with the metabolic syndrome, as well as for many patients with type 2 diabetes:

- Lopid (gemfibrozol)—a drug designed to lower triglycerides, but it is also associated with potentially serious side effects.

- Lipitor—a statin drug used to lower LDL cholesterol levels.

- Altace—an ACE inhibitor drug used in the treatment of high blood pressure.

- Avandia or Actos—potentially dangerous drugs (see page 191) used to lower blood sugar levels. Doctors prescribe these drugs because they are told that the drugs will help reduce the risk of atherosclerosis as well.

- Metformin (glucophage) is prescribed because doctors are told that it will reduce the risk of type 2 diabetes in patients with the metabolic syndrome. What the doctors don't know is that moderate exercise is twice as effective in achieving this goal (as discussed below).

- Nexium—an acid-blocker drug. It is often prescribed to deal with some of the gastrointestinal side effects produced by some of the other drugs.

Do these drugs really benefit the patients? That is highly debatable, given their side effects, interactions, and failure to address the real issues underlying metabolic syndrome as well as type 2 diabetes. Nonetheless, as the drug industry tries to expand its market, there is a tremendous push to get doctors to prescribe these multidrug regimens for all patients with metabolic syndrome and type 2 diabetes as early as possible.

OBESITY IS THE BIGGEST THREAT
TO AMERICA'S FUTURE

The drug industry and the conventional medical community have played a significant role in another serious epidemic in the United States—obesity.

Conventional Wisdom Once Again Proved Wrong

Patients with type 2 diabetes have been medicated in an attempt to achieve very tight control of blood sugar. It would seem to make sense that if you can improve the control of blood sugar levels, there will be a decrease in the complications of diabetes, and in mortality from diabetes. Although this practice became the unofficial gold standard of care, it had never been properly tested. That led the National Heart, Lung, and Blood Institute (NHLBI) to develop a study of approximately 10,000 patients with type 2 diabetes and either heart disease or two risk factors for heart disease. This study, named the ACCORD trial, was stopped prematurely because there was a higher rate of mortality from heart attacks in the patients being treated to achieve normal blood sugar control with a target for hemoglobin A_{1C} (HbA_{1C}, an indicator of blood sugar control) of less than 6 percent compared with those for whom the target was 7.0 percent to 7.9 percent.

Researchers and various medical experts scrambled to explain these results to the press, but the explanation seemed clear to me. To achieve the desired goal, these subjects were given higher dosages of drugs known to be associated with promoting heart disease. The results are not really surprising in light of the known issues with diabetes medications as well as some of the other drugs used in the trial (see the list on page 182 for an idea of what these patients were probably taking).

The drug companies offer their little pills for the treatment of diabetes, prediabetes, and metabolic syndrome in an attempt to overcome the effects of obesity, dietary excess, and an inactive lifestyle.

Each year obesity-related conditions cost more than $100 billion and cause an estimated 300,000 premature deaths in the United States. Although terrorism, environmental pollution, and dwindling natural resources certainly put the future of our nation in peril, a very strong case can be made that the obesity epidemic is the most significant threat to the future of the United States as well as other nations. In 1962, the proportion of obesity in America's population was at 13 percent. By 1980 it had risen to 15 percent, by 1994 to 23 percent, and by 2004 to one out of three, or 33 percent. Approximately 65 million adult Americans are now obese—more than the total populations of Britain, France, or Italy. And there is no end in sight. This trend is still rising rapidly. In particular, the percentage of children who are obese is rising at an alarming rate.

OBESITY AND HEALTH

Can you be healthy and fat? No. According to a recent study by the RAND organization, obesity is more damaging to health than smoking, high levels of alcohol consumption, and poverty.[2] Obesity affects all major bodily systems—heart, lungs, muscle, and bones. The health effects associated with obesity include, but are not limited to, the following:

- Metabolic syndrome—Approximately one-third of overweight or obese people in the United States have metabolic syndrome.

- High blood pressure—Additional fat tissue in the body needs oxygen and nutrients in order to live, so the blood vessels are required to circulate more blood to the fat tissue. This increases the work of the heart because it must pump more blood through additional blood vessels. More circulating blood also means more pressure on the artery walls. Higher pressure on the artery walls increases blood pressure. In addition, extra weight can raise the heart rate and reduce the body's ability to transport blood through the vessels.

- Diabetes—Obesity, particularly abdominal obesity, is the major cause of type 2 diabetes. Obesity can cause resistance to insulin, the hormone that regulates blood sugar. When obesity causes insulin resistance, the body's blood sugar level becomes elevated. Even moderate obesity dramatically increases the risk of diabetes.

- Heart disease—Atherosclerosis (hardening of the arteries) is present 10 times more often in obese people compared with those who are not obese. Coronary artery disease is also more prevalent because fatty deposits build up in arteries that supply the heart. Narrowed arteries and reduced blood flow to the heart can cause chest pain (angina) or a heart attack. Blood clots can also form in narrowed arteries and cause a stroke.

▸ Cancer—In women, being overweight contributes to an increased risk of various cancers, including cancer of the breast, colon, gallbladder, and uterus. Men who are overweight have a higher risk of colon and prostate cancers.

▸ Joint problems, including osteoarthritis—Obesity can affect the knees and hips because of the stress placed on the joints by extra weight. Joint replacement surgery is commonly performed on damaged joints, but it may not be an advisable option for an obese person, because the artificial joint has a higher risk of loosening and causing further damage.

▸ Sleep apnea and respiratory problems—Sleep apnea, a condition in which people stop breathing for brief periods, interrupts sleep throughout the night and causes sleepiness during the day. It also causes heavy snoring. Respiratory problems associated with obesity occur when added weight at the chest wall squeezes the lungs and restricts breathing. Sleep apnea is also associated with high blood pressure.

▸ Psychosocial effects—In a culture where the usual ideal of physical attractiveness is to be overly thin, people who are overweight or obese frequently suffer disadvantages. Overweight and obese persons are often blamed for their condition and may be considered lazy or weak-willed. It is not uncommon for overweight or obesity to result in having a lower income or in having few or no romantic relationships. Disapproval of overweight people may progress to bias, discrimination, and even torment.

Obesity Defined

The simplest definition of "obesity" is an excessive amount of body fat. Obesity is distinguishable from "overweight," which refers to an excess of body weight relative to height. A muscular athlete may be overweight yet have a low percentage of body fat. Given this distinction, it is obvious that using body weight alone as an index of obesity is not entirely accurate. Nonetheless, a simple measure known as body mass index (BMI) is now the accepted standard for classifying individuals with regard to body composition. The BMI generally correlates well with a person's total body fat. It is calculated by dividing a person's weight in kilograms by his or her height in meters squared. The mathematical formula is $weight/height^2$ or kg/m^2. You are not likely to actually calculate your BMI, so here is a simple table. To use the table, find the appropriate height in the left-hand column. Move across the row to the given weight. The number at the top of the column is the BMI for that height and weight.

Body Mass Index

BMI (kg/m²)	19	20	21	22	23	24	25	26	27	28	29	30	35	40
Height, inches	Weight, pounds													
58	91	96	100	105	110	115	119	124	129	134	138	143	167	191
59	94	99	104	109	114	119	124	128	133	138	143	148	173	198
60	97	102	107	112	118	123	128	133	138	143	148	153	179	204
61	100	106	111	116	122	127	132	137	143	148	153	158	185	211
62	104	109	115	120	126	131	136	142	147	153	158	164	191	218
63	107	113	118	124	130	135	141	146	152	158	163	169	197	225
64	110	116	122	128	134	140	145	151	157	163	169	174	204	232
65	114	120	126	132	138	144	150	156	162	168	174	180	210	240
66	118	124	130	136	142	148	155	161	167	173	179	186	216	247
67	121	127	134	140	146	153	159	166	172	178	185	191	223	255
68	125	131	138	144	151	158	164	171	177	184	190	197	230	262

BMI (kg/m²)	19	20	21	22	23	24	25	26	27	28	29	30	35	40
69	128	135	142	149	155	162	169	176	182	189	196	203	236	270
70	132	139	146	153	160	167	174	181	188	195	202	207	243	278
71	136	143	150	157	165	172	179	186	193	200	208	215	250	286
72	140	147	154	162	169	177	184	191	199	206	213	221	258	294
73	144	151	159	166	174	182	189	197	204	212	219	227	265	302
74	148	155	163	171	179	186	194	202	210	218	225	233	272	311
75	152	160	168	176	184	192	200	208	216	224	232	240	279	319
76	156	164	172	180	189	197	205	213	221	230	238	246	287	328

A BMI between 25 and 29.9 indicates overweight. Obesity is defined as a BMI of 30 or greater. To put BMI in perspective, a woman five feet four inches tall with a BMI of 30 is about 30 pounds above her ideal body weight. Obesity is not a matter of simply being a few pounds overweight. It reflects a significant amount of excess fat. There is one more calculation that is important—your waist size. The combination of your BMI and your waist circumference is very good indicator of your risk of all the diseases associated with obesity, especially the major killers: heart disease, stroke, cancer, and diabetes.

Risk of Associated Disease According to BMI and Waist Size

BMI	Classification	Waist Less Than or Equal to 40 Inches (Men) or 35 Inches (Women)	Waist Greater Than 40 Inches (men) or 35 Inches (women)
18.5 or less	Underweight	—	NA
18.5–24.9	Normal	—	NA
25.0–29.9	Overweight	Increased	High
30.0–34.9	Obese	High	Very high
35.0–39.9	Obese	Very high	Very high
40 or greater	Extremely obese	Extremely high	Extremely high

ABDOMINAL OBESITY—
A KEY COMPONENT OF
METABOLIC SYNDROME AND
INSULIN RESISTANCE

Abdominal obesity is highly associated with metabolic syndrome, insulin resistance, elevated inflammatory markers, high cholesterol, high triglycerides, high blood pressure, dyslipidemia, and hypertension. It is much more strongly linked to these conditions than body mass index is. So, apparently it is not how much you weigh, but rather where you store your fat, that determines your risk of cardiovascular disease.

Abdominal fat tissue was previously regarded as an inert storage depot; however, the emerging concept describes adipose tissue as a complex and highly active metabolic and endocrine organ. Fat cells secrete adipokines, hormonelike compounds that control insulin sensitivity and appetite. As abdominal fat accumulates, it leads to alterations in adipokines that ultimately promote insulin resistance and an increased appetite, thereby adding more abdominal fat. Fortunately, reduction of abdominal fat through dietary means and increased physical activity can reestablish insulin sensitivity and reduce appetite.

To determine your waist circumference, locate the upper hip bone and place a measuring tape around the abdomen (ensuring that the tape is horizontal). The tape should be snug but should not compress the skin. If your waist circumference is (for a man) greater than 40 inches or (for a woman) greater than 35 inches, there is no need to do any further calculation, as this measurement alone has been shown to be a major risk factor for both CVD and type 2 diabetes. If your waist circumference is less than these values, you need to determine your waist-to-hip ratio. To do this, measure the circumference of your waist as before and the circumference of your hips at the greatest protrusion of the buttocks. Divide the waist circumference by the hip circumference. A waist-to-hip ratio above 1.0 for men and above 0.8 for women increases the risk of developing CVD, type 2 diabetes, high blood pressure, and gout.

1. Measure the circumference of your waist: _____

2. Measure the circumference of your hips: _____

Divide the waist measurement by the hip measurement: waist/hip = _____
(this is your waist-to-hip ratio)

DIABETES—A MAJOR CONSEQUENCE OF OBESITY

Diabetes is one of the biggest drains on our society's resources—both financial and human. The total economic toll of diabetes in the United States alone is more than $100 billion dollars annually. To put this in perspective, the average annual cost of health care for a diabetic is approximately $12,000, whereas the cost for an adult without diabetes is about $3,000. Diabetes is responsible for more than 30 million visits to doctors each year, and for a total of about 15 million days of hospitalization for diabetes-related

---

A Diabetes Primer

Diabetes is divided into two major categories: type 1 and type 2. Type 1 diabetes is associated with complete destruction of the beta cells of the pancreas that manufacture the hormone insulin. Individuals with type 1 diabetes will require lifelong insulin to control blood sugar levels. About 5 to 10 percent of all diabetics are type 1.

In type 2 diabetes insulin levels are typically elevated, indicating a loss of sensitivity to insulin by the cells of the body. Approximately 90 percent of individuals categorized as having type 2 diabetes are obese. Obesity greatly reduces the sensitivity of cells to the hormone insulin.

Prediabetes is a condition that occurs when a person's blood glucose levels are higher than normal (>101 mg/dL), but not high enough for a diagnosis of type 2 diabetes (>126 mg/dL). There are almost as many people in the United States with prediabetes (about 16 million) as there are with type 2 diabetes (18 million).

issues. In addition to an earlier death, diabetes carries significant risks of serious complications such as blindness, a need for dialysis, and limb amputation.

The major complications of diabetes are as follows:

▸ Heart disease and stroke—Adults with diabetes have death rates from cardiovascular disease about two to four times higher than adults without diabetes.

▸ High blood pressure—About 75 percent of adults with diabetes have high blood pressure.

▸ Blindness—Diabetes is the leading cause of blindness among adults.

▸ Kidney disease—Diabetes is the leading reason why people need to go on dialysis, accounting for 43 percent of new cases.

▸ Nervous system disease—About 60 percent to 70 percent of people with diabetes have mild to severe nervous system damage. Severe forms of diabetic nerve disease are a major contributing cause of lower-extremity amputations.

▸ Amputations—More than 60 percent of lower-limb amputations in the United States occur among people with diabetes.

▸ Periodontal disease—Almost one-third of people with diabetes have severe periodontal (gum) disease.

▸ Pain—Many diabetics have chronic pain due to conditions such as arthritis, neuropathy, circulatory insufficiency, or muscle pain (fibromyalgia).

▸ Depression—This is a common accompaniment of diabetes. Clinical depression can often begin years before diabetes is fully evident, and it is difficult to treat in poorly controlled diabetics.

▸ Autoimmune disorders—Thyroid disease, inflammatory arthritis, and other diseases of the immune system commonly add to the suffering of diabetics.

DIABETES—WHAT THE DRUG COMPANIES WON'T TELL YOU AND YOUR DOCTOR DOESN'T KNOW

Type 2 diabetes is an entirely preventable disease, even if it's in your family. If you have type 2 diabetes, in most cases, you can eliminate the need for drugs and normalize blood sugar levels by achieving your ideal body weight. In Chapter 1, I stated that the current treatment of type 2 diabetes is absurd. The research is quite clear—oral medications to treat type 2 diabetes do not alter the long-term development of the disease. The drugs are quite effective in the short term, but they create a false sense of security and ultimately fail starting a vicious circle in which they are prescribed at higher dosages or in combination with other drugs, leading to increased mortality. That is right; the long-term use of these drugs is actually associated with an earlier death, compared with control groups of diabetics who are not being given the drugs. The major categories of these oral diabetes drugs are:

- ▸ Alpha-glucosidase inhibitors: acarbose (Precose); miglitol (Glyset)

- ▸ Sulfonylureas: acetohexamide (Dymelor); chlorpropamide (Diabinese, Insulase); glimepiride (Amaryl); glipizide (Glipizide, Glucotrol); glyburide (Diabeta, Micronase); repaglinide (Prandin); tolazamide (Tolinase); tolbutamide (Orinase)

- ▸ Biguanide type (non-sulfonylureas): metformin (Glucophage)

- ▸ Sulfonylurea/metformin combination: glyburide + metformin (Glucovance)

- ▸ Insulin-response enhancers: pioglitazone (Actos); rosiglitazone maleate (Avandia); troglitazone (Rezulin)

- ▸ Insulin-production enhancers: repaglinide (Prandin); nateglinide (Starlix)

The most widely prescribed of these drugs is metformin (Glucophage). Metformin is a drug with a profile that is generally more favorable than the other oral diabetes drugs for most type 2 diabetics requiring medication. Although studies have found that metformin alone shows a decrease in heart attacks and all diabetes-related deaths, it does not work at all in about 25 percent of cases and tends to lose its effectiveness over time.[3] When it does lose effectiveness, it is usually combined with a sulfonylurea. On their own, these drugs are of limited value, and there is some evidence that sulfonylureas actually have harmful long-term side effects. For example, in a famous study conducted by the University Group Diabetes Program (UDGP), it was shown that the rate of death due to a heart attack or stroke was 2.5 times greater in the group taking tolbutamide (a sulfonylurea) than in the group controlling type 2 diabetes by diet alone. Though newer sulfonylureas are considered safer than tolbutamide, there still remains considerable concern regarding their effects on the heart.[4] In addition, sulfonylureas promote weight gain, thereby fighting against the diabetic's necessary efforts to lose weight. The combination of metformin with glyburide or gliblencamide, like taking a sulfonylurea alone, actually increases premature mortality.[5]

The thiazolidinediones are the newest class of oral diabetes drugs. Like pioglitazone (Actose) and rosiglitazone (Avandia), these drugs appear to be extremely dangerous. The first drug in this class, Rezulin (troglitazone), was removed from the market because of widespread deaths due to liver failure. Pooled results from 42 different studies with Avandia found a 43 percent increase in the number of heart attacks and a 64 percent increased risk of dying from heart disease in patients taking it, compared with type 2 diabetics given a placebo.[6] In addition, both Actose and Avandia are also associated with significant weight gain. Although these drugs may have some benefits in lowering blood sugar levels, it is clear that the side effects outweigh the benefits.

PREVENTING DIABETES IN
HIGH-RISK INDIVIDUALS

Several large, well-designed trials have shown that lifestyle and dietary modifications can be used effectively to prevent type 2 diabetes. That fact has not dissuaded drug companies from sponsoring studies attempting to show prevention of diabetes with their drugs. The goal is to tap into the prediabetes market. Since there are almost as many Americans with prediabetes as with type 2 diabetes, drug companies can double their profits from oral diabetes drugs if they can persuade doctors to prescribe them for people with fasting blood sugar levels between 101 and 125 mg/dL (anything over 126 signifies diabetes). The drug companies are very quick to point out their drugs do seem to produce a preventive effect, but they fail to tell the doctors that the degree of prevention achieved by drugs pales in comparison with the effectiveness of diet and lifestyle. For example, consider one of the most celebrated studies. The drug companies' sales reps tell doctors that in this study metformin reduced the incidence of diabetes by 31 percent, but they fail to tell the doctors that walking for 30 minutes a day five days a week reduced the incidence by 58 percent.[7] Clearly, the lifestyle intervention was significantly more effective than metformin.

HUNGER-FREE FOREVER

The most important goal in the effective treatment of type 2 diabetes (as well as of metabolic syndrome and high blood pressure), in the overwhelming majority of cases, is achieving ideal body weight. To help in that goal, Dr. Michael Lyon and I developed the Hunger Free Forever plan to make effective, permanent weight loss a reality. Our program utilizes exciting scientific breakthroughs to stabilize blood sugar levels, improve the action of insulin, normalize appetite, and help people enjoy a high degree of satiety. This simple approach makes it easy to reach and maintain body weight goals.

Satiety is defined as the state of being full or gratified to the point of satisfaction. Research has shown that humans eat to achieve satiety and those who are overweight have more food cravings and resist satiety even after eating adequate amounts of food. Our program uncovers the reasons for these cravings and this resistance to satiety, and it provides keys to restoring normal appetite control. We have found it to be successful whether someone wants to lose five pounds or 200 pounds.

If you have struggled to achieve your ideal body weight, if you have tried various diets only to end up weighing more than when you started, if you feel that when you simply look at food it magically winds up on your thighs, or if you always feel hungry and never feel satisfied, then I strongly encourage you to read our book *Hunger Free Forever* for detailed information. But to get started, please see Appendix C, The Hunger Free Forever Program.

Soft Drinks Linked to Metabolic Syndrome

The frequent consumption of soft drinks, whether regular or diet, is associated with obesity and increased risk of metabolic syndrome and diabetes. A team of researchers at Harvard analyzed consumption of soft drinks in more than 6,000 individuals participating in the Framingham Heart Study.[8] Their results are astounding. Drinking one or more soft drinks per day was associated with several conditions.

Component of the metabolic syndrome	Increased risk
Increased waist circumference	30%
Elevated blood sugar	25%
High blood pressure ($\geq$ 135/85 mm Hg or on treatment)	18%
High triglycerides	25%
Low HDL cholesterol	32%
Overall incidence of metabolic syndrome	44%

Presumably individuals who drink soda, with sugar or without, tend to have a greater intake of calories, consume more saturated and trans fats, consume less fiber, and have a more sedentary lifestyle. And, despite the fact that diet soda has zero calories, the findings are not entirely surprising, because previous studies on diet soft drinks have linked them to weight gain and high blood pressure. Diet sodas are thought to lead to a stronger dietary preference for sweeter foods, as well as to disrupt appetite control.

HIGH BLOOD PRESSURE

Each time the heart beats, it sends blood coursing through the arteries. The peak reading of the pressure exerted by this contraction is the systolic pressure. Between beats the heart relaxes, and blood pressure drops. This lower reading is referred to as the diastolic pressure. Blood pressure readings are in millimeters (mm) of mercury (Hg). A normal blood pressure reading for adults is 120 (systolic)/80 (diastolic). Readings above this level are a major risk factor for heart attack and stroke. High blood pressure can be divided into the following categories:

Prehypertension (120–139/80–89)

Borderline (120–160/90–94)

Mild (140–160/95–104)

Moderate 140–180/105–114)

Severe (160+/115+)

More than 80 percent of patients with high blood pressure are in the borderline-to-moderate range. Because most of these cases can be brought under control through changes in diet and lifestyle, it can be concluded that 80 percent of the prescriptions for high blood pressure are ill-advised. In fact, in comparisons of cases of borderline to mild hypertension, many non-drug therapies such as diet, exercise, and relaxation have proved superior to drugs. Here is another important point: several well-designed long-term clinical studies found that people taking diuretics, beta-blockers, or both not only experienced unnecessary side effects, but also had an increased risk of heart disease. Keep in mind that the reason why high blood pressure is treated is to reduce the risk of heart disease and strokes. Although the newer classes of drugs, the calcium channel blockers and angiotensin-converting enzyme (ACE) inhibitors, appear to be safer and to have fewer side effects, they are also not without problems.

ANTIHYPERTENSIVE DRUGS

The four major categories of drugs that lower blood pressure are diuretics, beta-blockers, calcium channel blockers, and ACE inhibitors. Here is a brief description of each drug, followed by current recommendations for the drug treatment of high blood pressure.

Diuretics

To lower blood pressure, diuretics reduce the volume of fluid in the blood and body tissues by promoting the elimination of salt and water through increased urination. In addition, diuretics also work to relax the smaller arteries of the body, allowing them to expand and increase the total fluid capacity of the arterial system. The net result of diuretics is lower pressure due to reduced volume in an expanded space. Thiazide diuretics are by far the most popular type—they are often the first drug used in treating mild to moderate high blood pressure. Examples of thiazide diuretics include:

- bendroflumethiazide (Naturetin)

- benzthiazide (Exna, Hydrex)

- chlorothiazide (Diuril); chlorthalidone (Hydone, Hygroton, Novo-Thalidone, Thalitone, Uridon); cyclothiazide (Anhydron)

- hydrochlorothiazide (Apo-Hydro, Diuchlor H, Esidrix, Hydro-chlor, HydroDIURIL, Neo-Codema, Novo-Hydrazide, Oretic, Urozide)

- hydroflumethiazide (Diucardin, Saluron)

- methyclothiazide (Aquatensen, Duretic, Enduron)

- metolazone (Diulo, Mykrox, Zaroxolyn)

- polythiazide (Renese)

- quinethazone (Hydromox)

- trichlormethiazide (Aquazide, Diurese, Metahydrin, Naqua, Trichlorex)

Some of the side effects of thiazide diuretics are light-headedness, higher blood sugar levels, higher uric acid levels, aggravation of gout, and muscle weakness and cramps caused by low potassium levels. Decreased libido and impotence are also reported. Less frequent side effects include allergic reactions, headaches, blurred vision, nausea, vomiting, and diarrhea.

Thiazide diuretics also cause a loss of potassium, magnesium, and calcium from the body. All these minerals have been shown to lower blood pressure and prevent heart attacks. The drugs also raise cholesterol and triglyceride levels; increase the viscosity of the blood; raise uric acid levels; and increase the stickiness of the platelets, making them likely to aggregate and form clots. All these factors may explain why thiazide diuretics may actually increase the risk of dying from a heart attack or stroke. Thiazide diuretics also have a tendency to worsen blood sugar control, so they are difficult to use safely with diabetics.

Beta-Blockers

Beta-blockers produce a reduced rate and force of contraction of the heart, as well as relaxing the arteries. In addition to high blood pressure, beta-blockers are also used in treating angina and certain rhythm disturbances of the heart. Because heart function is reduced with beta-blockers, there is a decreased need for oxygen and angina is relieved. In the long term, however, this inhibition of heart function can lead to heart failure. Beta-blockers have fallen out of favor because they are not effective in reducing cardiovascular mortality, and they have been shown to increase the risk of developing diabetes by about 30 percent.

Beta-blockers produce some significant side effects in many patients. Because cardiac output is reduced in a more relaxed arterial system, it is often difficult to get enough blood and oxygen to the hands, feet, and brain. This results in the typical symptoms described by users of beta-blockers, such as cold hands and feet, nerve tingling, impaired mental function, fatigue, dizziness, depression, lethargy, reduced libido, and impotence. Beta-blockers also raise cholesterol and triglyceride levels considerably. This may explain some of the negative effects in the clinical studies, which failed to demonstrate any significant benefit of beta-blockers in reducing mortality due to cardiovascular disease.

It is extremely important not to discontinue a beta-blocker suddenly. Stopping this medication suddenly can produce a withdrawal syndrome consisting of headache, increased heart rate, and a dramatic increase in blood pressure.

Examples of beta-blockers include:

- acebutolol (Acebutolol, Sectral)

- atenolol (Atenolol, Senormin, Tenormin)

- bisoprolol fumarate (Zebeta)

- carteolol (Cartrol, Ocupress)

- metoprolol succinate (Toprol-XL)

- metoprolol tartrate (Lopressor)

- nadolol (Corgard)

- penbutolol sulfate (Levatol)

- pindolol (Visken)

- propranolol (Betachron, Inderal, Pronol)

- timolol maleate (Blocadren, Timoptic)

Calcium Channel Blockers

Calcium channel blockers, along with ACE inhibitors, have taken over the top spots in the drug treatment of high blood pressure because they are better tolerated than diuretics and beta-blockers. Although calcium channel blockers have been shown to lower the risk of stroke, they carry the same increased risk for heart attacks as the older approach (diuretics and beta-blockers).

Calcium channel blockers work (as the term implies) by blocking the normal passage of calcium through certain channels in cell walls. Since calcium is required in the function of nerve transmission and muscle contraction, the effect of blocking the calcium channel is to slow down nerve conduction and inhibit the contraction of the muscle. In the heart and vascular system, this action results in reducing the rate and force of contraction, relaxing the arteries, and slowing the nerve impulses in the heart.

Although they are much better tolerated than beta-blockers and diuretics, calcium channel blockers still produce some mild side effects, including constipation, allergic reactions, fluid retention, dizziness, headache, fatigue, and impotence (in about 20 percent of users). More serious side effects include disturbances of heart rate or function, heart failure, and angina.

Examples of calcium channel blockers include:

- amlodipine (Norvasc)

- diltiazem (Cardizem CD, Cartia, Dilacor Xr, Diltia Xt, Tiazac)

- felodipine (Plendil)

- lacidipine (Motens)

- lercanidipine (Zanidip)

- nicardipine (Cardene, Carden SR)

- nifedipine (Adalat CC, Procardia XL)

- nimodipine (Nimotop)

- nisoldipine (Sular)

- nitrendipine (Cardif, Nitrepin)

- verapamil (Calan, Covera-Hs, Isoptin, Verelan)

Angiotension-Converting Enzyme (ACE) Inhibitors

The ACE inhibitors prevent the formation of angiotensin II, a substance that increases both the fluid volume and the degree of constriction of the blood vessels. An ACE inhibitor relaxes the arterial walls and reduces fluid volume. Unlike the beta-blockers and calcium channel blockers, however,

ACE inhibitors actually improve heart function and increase blood and oxygen flow to the heart, liver, and kidneys. This effect may explain why ACE inhibitors are the only antihypertensive drugs that appear to reduce the risk of heart attacks. Unfortunately, they do not reduce the risk of strokes.

The newer ACE inhibitors are generally well tolerated but have many of the same side effects as the other antihypertensives, including dizziness, light-headedness, and headache. The most common side effect is a dry nighttime cough. The ACE inhibitors can also cause potassium buildup and kidney problems, so potassium levels and kidney function must be monitored.

Examples of ACE inhibitors include:

- benazepril (Lotensin)

- captopril (Capoten)

- captopril/hydrochlorothizaide (Capozide)

- enalapril maleate (Vasotec, Renitec)

- fosinopril sodium (Monopril)

- lisinopril (Lisodur, Lopril, Novatec Prinivil, Zestril)

- perindopril (Coversyl, Aceon)

- quinapril/magnesium carbonate (Accupril)

- ramipril (Altace, Tritace, Ramace, Ramiwin)

- trandolapril (Mavik)

Current Drug Treatment of High Blood Pressure
For many years the drug of first choice for high blood pressure was a thiazide diuretic alone or in combination with a beta-blocker. As mentioned earlier, because of a lack of effectiveness in reducing the cardiovascular death rate, and because of side effects noted in numerous studies, this approach has somewhat fallen out of favor. Currently, the most commonly used medication is a diuretic alone or in combination with newer medica-

tions designed to relax the arteries, such as calcium channel blockers and ACE inhibitors.

A diuretic or any of these other drugs alone is referred to as a "step 1" drug. Thiazide diuretics are still the most popular step 1 drug but may soon be displaced by calcium channel blockers or ACE inhibitors. Beta-blockers are not suitable as step 1 drugs, owing to their known side effects. A step 2 approach uses two medications; a step 3 approach uses three; and a step 4 approach uses four. Physicians are instructed to use single therapies before using combinations of medicines. Of course, they are also instructed to utilize nondrug therapies first, but that rarely occurs.

HIGH BLOOD PRESSURE—
A RATIONAL APPROACH

Although medical textbooks state that the cause is unknown in 95 percent of cases, hypertension is closely related to lifestyle and dietary factors, which have a direct effect on the health of the arteries. Important lifestyle factors that may cause high blood pressure include stress, lack of exercise, and smoking. Dietary factors include obesity; a high sodium-to-potassium ratio; a low-fiber, high-sugar diet; high intake of saturated fat; low intake of omega-3 fatty acid; and a diet low in calcium, magnesium, and vitamin C. These same factors are also known to promote hardening of the arteries (atherosclerosis) and impair the ability of the kidneys to regulate fluid volume and control blood pressure. In addition, it is important to rule out heavy metal toxicity as an underlying factor in high blood pressure (see Chapter 2 for more information).

Achieving ideal body weight is the most important dietary recommendation for those with high blood pressure. However, overweight people who lose even a modest amount of weight experience a reduction in blood pressure that can significantly reduce the need for antihypertensive drugs.

Dietary Approaches to Stop Hypertension

Two very large studies have shown quite clearly that diet can be effective in lowering blood pressure. These studies, the Dietary Approaches to Stop Hypertension (DASH), tested a diet that was rich in fruits, vegetables, and low-fat dairy foods, and low in saturated and total fat. The first study showed that a diet rich in fruits, vegetables, and low-fat dairy products can reduce blood pressure in the general population and in people with hypertension.[9] To be effective, the original DASH diet did not require either sodium restriction or weight loss—the two traditional dietary tools to control blood pressure. The second study from the DASH research group found that combining the original DASH diet with sodium restriction is more effective than either the DASH diet or sodium restriction alone.[10]

In the first trial, the DASH diet produced a net blood pressure reduction of 11.4 and 5.5 mm Hg systolic and diastolic, respectively, in patients with hypertension. In the second trial, sodium intake was also restricted. The most common form of sodium is sodium chloride, which is table salt (Fast foods; processed meats, such as bacon, sausage, and ham; and canned soups and vegetables are all examples of foods that are generally very high in sodium.)

Many studies have shown varying success rates with a sodium-restricted diet in the treatment of high blood pressure, but the DASH diet with the lower sodium level led to a mean systolic blood pressure that was 11.5 mm Hg lower in participants with hypertension. These results are clinically significant and indicate that a sodium intake below 1,500 mg daily can lower blood pressure significantly and quickly. As a point of reference, 1 teaspoon of table salt contains 2,300 mg of sodium.

The reason why many studies using sodium restriction alone failed to lower blood pressure is that in order to be effective sodium restriction must be accompanied by a high potassium intake.[11] Since the best way to boost potassium levels is to increase the intake of fruits and vegetables, that may explain why the results were so good in the second DASH study. Most Americans have a potassium-to-sodium ratio of less than 1:2, meaning that they ingest twice as much sodium as potassium. For optimal health, the research indicates that we should be consuming five times as much potassium as sodium (5:1). The easiest way to achieve this ratio is to avoid prepared foods and table salt, and to use potassium chloride salt substitutes, such as

Avoid Junk Food and Hidden Sources of Empty Calories

According to the third National Health and Nutrition Examination Survey, which studied eating habits among 15,000 American adults, one-third of the average diet in this country is made up of unhealthy foods, including potato chips, crackers, salted snack foods, candy, gum, fried fast food, and soft drinks. These items offer little in terms of protein, vitamins, or minerals. But they do have lots of empty calories in the form of sugar and fat. Here are guidelines for making healthier eating choices:

▶ Read labels carefully. If sugar, fat, or salt is one of the first three ingredients listed, the product is probably not a good option.

▶ Be aware that certain words appearing on a label—such as sucrose, glucose, maltose, lactose, fructose, corn syrup, or white grape juice concentrate—mean that sugar has been added.

▶ Look not just at the percentage of calories from fat, but also the number of grams of fat. For every 5 grams (g) of fat in a serving, you are eating the equivalent of 1 teaspoon of fat.

▶ If a snack doesn't provide at least 2 g of fiber, it's not a good choice.

▶ Keep an eye on the sodium content. If a package lists more than 10 percent of your total sodium allowance per serving, the product is not a good choice.

the popular brands NoSalt® and Nu-Salt®, instead. You can find these products right next to the sodium chloride salts at your local grocery or health food store.

Special foods for people with high blood pressure include celery; garlic and onions to lower cholesterol; nuts and seeds, or their oils, for their essential fatty acid content; cold-water fish such as salmon and mackerel, or fish oil products concentrated for the omega-3 fatty acids EPA and DHA; green leafy vegetables and sea vegetables for their calcium and magnesium; whole flaxseeds, whole grains, and legumes for their fiber; and foods rich in vitamin C, such as broccoli and citrus fruits.

Other Recommendations to Lower Blood Pressure

Caffeine, alcohol, and tobacco should be eliminated. Stress reduction techniques, such as biofeedback, meditation, yoga, deep breathing exercises, and regular aerobic exercise may offer some benefit in lowering blood pressure without the use of drugs. For example, RESPeRATE is a computerized biofeedback device approved by the FDA for reducing stress and lowering blood pressure. It works by analyzing your breathing pattern to create a personalized melody that it transmits to earphones. The goal is to synchronize your breathing to the melody that you hear through the earphones—about 10 breaths a minute, with particularly long exhalations. The theory behind RESPeRATE is that many people with high blood pressure have increased activity of the sympathetic nervous system—the part of your nervous system that controls blood flow. Slow, deep breathing reduces this activity, allowing blood pressure to return to normal. Studies of people with high blood pressure who use RESPeRATE as directed report an average decrease in blood pressure of 14 mm Hg. For more information, see RESPeRATE (www.resperate.com)

The most effective natural product for lowering blood pressure is a purified mixture of small peptides (proteins) derived from muscle of the fish bonito (a member of the tuna family). Basically, these peptides work to lower blood pressure by inhibiting ACE (angiotensin converting enzyme). This enzyme converts angiotensin I to angiotensin II, which is a compound that increases both the fluid volume and the degree of constriction of the blood vessels. If we use a garden hose as a model to illustrate the pressure in your arteries, the formation of angiotensin II would be similar to pinching off the hose while turning up the faucet full blast. When the formation of this compound is inhibited, anti-ACE peptides relax the arterial walls and reduce fluid volume. Anti-ACE peptides exert the strongest inhibition of ACE reported for any naturally occurring substance available.

Three clinical studies have shown that anti-ACE peptides from bonito (daily dosage 1,500 mg) significantly lower blood pressure in people with high blood pressure (hypertension).[12] Anti-ACE peptides appear to be effective in about two-thirds of people with high blood pressure—about the same percentage as many prescription drugs, but without the side effects.

The degree of to which blood pressure was reduced in these studies was quite significant; typically, pressure was reduced systolic by at least 10 mm Hg and diastolic pressure by 7 mm Hg in people with prehypertension and borderline hypertension. Greater reductions will be seen in people with higher initial blood pressure readings.

Anti-ACE peptides do not appear to produce any side effects, according to human safety studies. The typical daily dosage is 1.5 grams (g), but even at a daily dosage of 30 g not a single subject in safety studies experienced any side effect—not even the dry nighttime cough so typical with the ACE inhibitor drugs.

THE IMPORTANCE OF SLEEP

No one would disagree that sleep is absolutely critical to human health; after all, sleep is the period of time when the body and mind are recharged. But does the quality of sleep have anything to do with the likelihood of developing obesity, type 2 diabetes, or high blood pressure? According to recent scientific studies, the answer is definitely yes.[13, 14, 15, 16] Sleep plays a prominent role in regulating hormones, including the hormones that in turn regulate blood sugar levels. Sleep deprivation has been shown to lead to impaired insulin action and multiple metabolic disturbances consistent with obesity and type 2 diabetes. It now appears that in addition to causing daytime drowsiness, mood and memory disturbances, impotence, and car wrecks, sleep disorders also promote insulin resistance and cardiovascular disease. In case you missed it, see page 175 for Seven Tips for a Good Night's Sleep.

The sleep disorder that is especially stressful to mechanisms controlling blood sugar is sleep apnea (characterized by brief interruptions of breathing during sleep), but even snoring is linked to poor blood sugar control. In an analysis of data from 70,000 female nurses followed for 10 years, occasional snoring was associated with a 41 percent increase and regular snoring was associated with a twofold (100 percent) increase in the frequency of developing type 2 diabetes. This increased risk occurred irrespective of body weight, indicating that snoring is an independent risk factor for type 2 diabetes.[17]

NASAL STRIPS, THROAT SPRAYS, AND SURGICAL OPTIONS TO RELIEVE SNORING

If you have watched a professional football game anytime since the mid-1990s you probably noticed that many of the players wear nasal strips. These adhesive strips mechanically open the nasal passages. The most popular brand is Breathe Right®. The strips were invented by Bruce Johnson in 1991. Bruce had always had trouble breathing through his nose, especially at night. Besides suffering from an array of allergies, Bruce has a deviated septum, a structural abnormality of the nose that constricts airflow through one nostril. This combination left his nose chronically congested and made sleeping through the night quite difficult. Lying in bed one night in 1988, he wondered, "Why not try opening the nasal passages mechanically from the outside of the nose?" His answer, after three years of development, took the form of a spring-loaded adhesive strip that he placed across the bridge of his nose to open it up. The device relieved his congestion and improved his sleep quality dramatically. He soon received a patent for his invention, and he brought his product to market in 1992.

Since that time, several clinical studies have confirmed what Bruce experienced himself—dilating the nasal passages can dramatically improve sleep quality and relieve snoring.[18, 19] However, this is not a cure-all. A variety of factors can contribute to snoring—body weight, alcohol, smoking, sleeping on your back, age, climate, and allergies—but the most common causes are related to airflow disruption through the nose, the throat, or both.

In the clinical studies, about half of the subjects experienced a significant benefit, but the other half did not. These results led to the development of Breathe Right® Throat Spray, a product designed to help people who snore as a result not of impaired nasal airflow but rather of loose tissue in the throat. This natural product contains an essential oil blend from wintergreen, peppermint, anise, and clove oil that tightens the throat tissue and reduces irritation. It seems to help many snorers sleep better. Some people experience the best results when they use both products. For more information on these products, see www.breatheright.com.

For severe snoring due to airway disruption through the throat, ultrasound-assisted uvulopalatoplasty appears to be a good option. It has replaced other surgical techniques because it has produced better results with fewer complications, such as bleeding or charring (the latter occurs with the use of lasers or electrosurgery). The procedure involves the use of sound waves to basically damage the tissue of the back of the throat, causing excessive soft tissue from the back of the throat and from the palate (the roof of the mouth separating the mouth from the nasal cavity) to tighten up and eliminate the loose tissue that causes snoring or sleep apnea in many people.

SLEEP APNEA MUST BE TREATED

First described in 1965, sleep apnea owes its name to a Greek word, *apnea*, meaning "want of breath." The pauses in breathing are almost always accompanied by snoring between apnea episodes, although not everyone who snores has this condition. Sleep apnea can also be characterized by choking sensations. The frequent interruptions of deep, restorative sleep often lead to excessive daytime sleepiness and may be associated with an early-morning headache. Approximately 18 million Americans are thought to suffer from sleep apnea.

Early recognition and treatment of sleep apnea are important because this condition is associated not only with an increased risk of obesity, type 2 diabetes, and high blood pressure, but also with severe daytime fatigue, irregular heartbeat, heart attack, and stroke, as well as a loss of memory and other intellectual capabilities. For many patients with sleep apnea, their bed partners or family members are the first to suspect that something is wrong, usually from the patients' heavy snoring and apparent struggle to breathe. Coworkers or friends may notice that a patient falls asleep during the day at inappropriate times (such as while driving a car, working, or talking). The patients themselves usually do not know they have a problem and may not believe it when told. It is important for them to see a doctor if they snore heavily or if a sleep partner has noticed periods of interrupted breathing during sleep. Sleep apnea should also be considered in anyone with significant daytime drowsiness or changes in intellectual function. Sleep apnea can be properly diagnosed only by a sleep disorder specialist and usually only in a sleep laboratory. Home testing equipment may also be provided through a sleep disorder specialist. The American Academy of Sleep Medicine (www .aasmnet.org) certifies specialists and sleep laboratories and, if appropriate, a referral to one of these centers should be sought from your physician.

Sleep apnea is most often caused when an excess amount of fatty tissue accumulates in the airway and causes it to be narrowed. With a narrowed airway, the person continues his or her efforts to breathe, but air cannot easily flow into or out of the nose or mouth. This narrowing of the airways results in heavy snoring, periods of no breathing, and frequent arousals (causing abrupt changes from deep sleep to light sleep). Ingestion of alcohol and sleeping pills increases the frequency and duration of breathing pauses in people with sleep apnea. In some cases sleep apnea occurs even if no airway obstruction or snoring is present. This form of sleep apnea is called central sleep apnea and is caused by a loss of perfect control over breathing by the brain. In both obstructive and central sleep apnea, obesity is the major risk factor and weight loss is the most important aspect of long-term management. People with sleep apnea experience periods of anoxia (oxygen deprivation of the brain), with each episode ending in arousal and a reinitiation of breathing. Seldom does the sufferer awaken enough to be aware of the problem. However, the combination of frequent periods of oxygen deprivation (20 to several hundreds of times per night) and the greatly disturbed sleep can greatly diminish the quality of life and lead to some very serious problems, including diabetes! Sleep apnea needs to be taken seriously, and it should always be treated.

Weight loss is also a critical part of the successful management of sleep apnea. Beyond that, the most common treatment of sleep apnea is the use of nasal continuous positive airway pressure (CPAP). In this procedure, the patient wears a mask over the nose during sleep, and pressure from an air blower forces air through the nasal passages. The air pressure is adjusted so that it is just enough to prevent the throat from collapsing during sleep. The pressure is constant and continuous. Nasal CPAP prevents airway closure while in use, but apnea episodes return when CPAP is stopped or if it is used improperly. The CPAC equipment is readily available and can be obtained with a doctor's prescription. It takes quite a while to get used to CPAP, but this method usually works well. In fact, I have had many patients who feel that they have been given a new lease on life with it.

Sleep Deprivation and Weight Gain

Sleep deprivation increases hunger and slows down metabolism, thereby promoting weight gain. The underlying mechanisms include:

► Increasing the level of cortisol, thereby promoting increased appetite, a craving for sugar, and weight gain. An elevated cortisol level also interferes with proper utilization of carbohydrates, leading to an increase in the storage of body fat and insulin resistance, a critical step in the development of obesity and diabetes.

► Elevating ghrelin and reducing leptin. Ghrelin is an appetite-stimulating hormone released mostly by the stomach. When ghrelin levels are up, people feel hungry. Leptin is a hormone, released by fat cells, that promotes a feeling of satiety.

In population studies, a dose-response relationship between short sleep duration and high body mass index (BMI) has been reported across all age groups. This observation alone indicates that sleeping more may help with weight loss. A very detailed analysis from the Wisconsin Sleep Cohort Study, a large sleep study that has been going on in Wisconsin for more than 15 years, provides even more insight.[20] The participants have been filling out questionnaires about their sleep habits, have kept sleep diaries, and have occasionally spent a night in the laboratory, where researchers studied their sleep in more detail. After sleeping overnight in the laboratory, the participants gave blood samples, which were tested for levels of leptin and ghrelin. What the researchers found is that habitual or acute short sleep duration produces low leptin and high ghrelin levels, a powerful recipe for an increased appetite and for a craving for carbohydrate-rich foods, including cake, candy, ice cream, pasta, and bread.

FINAL COMMENTS

My key point in this chapter is that drugs cannot compensate for the effects of diet and lifestyle. Diabetes and high blood pressure are very serious conditions that must not be ignored. Unfortunately, treatment with current drugs simply provides drug companies with very good customers for a relatively long time. Remember that the main goal is achieving ideal body weight. To help you with that goal, I recommend following the Hunger Free Forever program described in this chapter and detailed in Appendix C. Beyond that, I recommend several dietary, lifestyle, and supplement strategies designed to help improve the action of insulin and normalize blood sugar levels. These recommendations are detailed thoroughly in *How to Prevent and Treat Diabetes with Natural Medicine* (which I cowrote with Dr. Lyon). This book is a source of information and guidance for anyone with either type 1 or type 2 diabetes. Appendix D on page 285 provides additional information and a summary of recommendations for individuals with metabolic syndrome, diabetes, and high blood pressure.

Regular physical exercise is an especially important therapy for metabolic syndrome, type 2 diabetes, and obesity. In fact, there are considerable data to show that physical inactivity is a major cause underlying these conditions. It is especially important to include exercise in a weight loss program, for the following factors:

▸ Exercise increases the sensitivity of our cells to insulin.

▸ When weight loss is achieved by dieting without exercise, a substantial portion of the total weight loss comes from lean tissue, primarily as loss of water.

▸ When exercise is included in a weight loss program, there is usually an improvement in body composition due to a gain in lean body weight, and in turn to an increase in muscle mass and a decrease in body fat.

▸ Exercise helps counter the reduction in basal metabolic rate (BMR) that usually accompanies dieting alone.

▸ Exercise increases BMR for an extended period of time following the exercise session.

▸ Moderate to intense exercise may have a suppressing effect on the appetite.

▸ People who exercise during and after weight reduction are better able to maintain the weight loss than those who do not exercise.

10

LOOKING BEHIND THE HEADLINES AND THROUGH THE BIAS

"Whoever controls the media—
the images—controls the culture."
—Allen Ginsberg

MANY AMERICANS ARE UNAWARE that prior to 1997 it was illegal for drug companies to advertise directly to consumers. Drug companies last year spent more than $6 billion advertising to consumers, and these ads resulted in an increase of more than 30 million prescriptions. Because of the continued success of direct-to-consumer advertising (despite the fact that most ads disclose side effects), you can expect even more such ads this year.

Over the years many of us in the natural health field have seen the media continue to disseminate questionable results from research studies in major medical journals and to hold these up as "proof" that the public is being duped into spending money on worthless natural products. (Interestingly, positive studies on natural products do not seem to receive nearly as much attention from the media. I hope this is not because drug companies are among their leading advertisers.) Of course, those of us who are knowledgeable about the merits of natural products try to mobilize our resources to counteract the negative statements, but this is often difficult when we are up against a research article published in a respected journal like the *New England Journal of Medicine, Lancet, British Medical Journal,* or *Journal of the*

American Medical Association (JAMA). Such journals are seemingly more credible than even the most reputable organizations, companies, and experts in the natural product industry.

THE SAW PALMETTO STORY

To illustrate my point, let's take a quick look at a recent double-blind study, which the media presented as evidence that saw palmetto extract does not relieve the symptoms of benign prostatic hyperplasia (BPH). This study was published in the *New England Journal of Medicine*.[1] The news releases that ensued included a report by the Associated Press that the "popular herbal pill used by millions of men doesn't reduce the frequent urge to go to the bathroom or other annoying symptoms of an enlarged prostate." That is not true at all. I have been writing about the benefits of saw palmetto extract in the treatment of BPH for more than 20 years. In my major publications on the subject I have pointed out that the success of saw palmetto extract is most obvious in the early stages of BPH, i.e., in mild to moderate cases. Most natural products are simply not powerful enough to overcome a disease in its advanced stages: e.g., this is true of ginkgo biloba extract for severe Alzheimer's disease, CoQ10 for severe heart failure, and Saint-John's-wort for severe depression. Nonetheless, by studying cases of severely advanced disease researchers seem to want to set the stage for a situation in which no observable effect can be seen with natural products. That is exactly how this study of BPH was designed: it was conducted with men who had severe cases.

This study of saw palmetto extract tells us only that it is important to use the extract early in the disease process. The study tells us nothing new, because detailed double-blind studies have clearly shown that roughly 90 percent of men with mild to moderate BPH experience improvement in symptoms during the first four to six weeks after starting saw palmetto extract: 320 milligrams (mg) per day of the liposterolic extract.[2, 3] The key is to start saw palmetto as soon as symptoms of BPH appear. (The symptoms include progressive urinary frequency and urgency; increased nighttime urination; hesitancy and intermittency; and reduced force and caliber of urine.)

If a man waits until his prostate has enlarged so much that it results in significant obstruction of the bladder, saw palmetto is not likely to work. But if he starts saw palmetto early enough, it actually works at least as effectively as popular prescription drugs, without the side effects. Perhaps that is what makes the drug companies nervous. Presumably, the drug companies are upset because more than 2 million men in the United States use saw palmetto extract instead of drugs to control the symptoms of BPH.

SOME "FISHY" MISINFORMATION

In early April 2006, there was another blatant misinformation campaign when headlines in the media claimed "Fish Oil Supplements Have No Effect on Heart Disease or Cancer." The source of this false statement was a review article published in the *British Medical Journal (BMJ)*.[4] What the study concluded and what the media grabbed hold of was this: "Long chain and shorter chain omega 3 fats do not have a clear effect on total mortality, combined cardiovascular events, or cancer." That is far different from what the study actually found. According to the lead author of the study, Dr. Lee Hooper:[5]

> We did not report that "long chain omega-3 does not offer any protection from heart disease," that "omega-3 fats have no effect on total mortality, combined cardiovascular events, or cancer" or that omega 3 fats are of "no benefit"—this is not what we found, or what we reported (despite our being misquoted in much of the press).

So, what was the truth behind the headline? Read on. But before you do, I want to stress that a high-quality fish oil supplement is one of the most important tools in the prevention and treatment of many diseases. That fact is irrefutable and is based on a large body of clinical evidence from double-blind, placebo-controlled trials. What Dr. Hooper and her group actually found by looking at the data was that taking omega-3 fatty acid was associated with a 13 percent reduction in mortality in study participants.

I do have some issues with this study, however. First, it was not a new study, but rather a detailed review and meta-analysis. The authors of a meta-analysis review the medical literature and then apply certain criteria to select published studies to include in their analysis. As a result, a meta-analysis is only as good as the studies it includes. If all the studies are of high quality and well designed, a meta-analysis can be quite helpful, because the total number of subjects is often greatly increased and that increase leads to greater statistical significance. However, if the meta-analysis includes a very large poorly designed study, it can tip the scales toward a wrong conclusion. That appears to be exactly what happened in this particular meta-analysis. Dr. Hooper's group included a study (the DART-2 study) that has been judged by the U.S. Department of Health and Human Services and various experts as having an extremely poor design.[6] One of the most serious problems was that the dietary instructions were given only at the start of the nine-year study and again after six months. People were simply told to eat more fish, but there was never any real verification that the subjects actually complied. If this single study is excluded (as it should have been), the results would have shown dramatically that fish oils are quite protective against cancer, heart disease, and strokes.

Another huge problem with the meta-analysis is that many of the studies utilized based the intake of omega-3 fatty acids on dietary, or "food frequency," questionnaires—which have been sharply criticized because they are often inaccurate. Researchers who have relied instead on blood measurements of the long-chain omega-3 fatty acids EPA and DHA have found that these are very clearly associated with a reduction in heart attacks and strokes. For example, the group with the highest intake of EPA and DHA had an 80 percent reduced risk of a fatal heart attack relative to the group with the lowest intake.[7] Obviously, that is a major reduction.

Another issue arises when the effects of fish are linked to the effects of long-chain omega-3 fatty acids. Fish is the best natural source of the long-chain omega-3 fatty acids, but our fish supply is also tainted with mercury, lead, pesticide residues, and other harmful compounds. Mercury has been known to increase the risk of cardiovascular disease. Although fish oils may protect against heart disease, is the benefit of eating fish worth a higher intake of mercury? Apparently not, as it has been shown that even though higher body levels of EPA and DHA were associated with a decreased risk of heart attacks, the higher the body mercury level the greater the risk of a heart attack.[8] Researchers have concluded that the high mercury content of fish may diminish the protective effect of fish against heart disease. So, it is entirely inappropriate to lump consumption of fish into an analysis of the health benefits of long-chain omega-3 fatty acids.

A pharmaceutical-grade fish oil supplement is part of the foundation for good health. In fact, the development of high-quality fish oil products is one of the major achievements of nutritional medicine. According to the totality of research, in order to significantly promote health and reduce the risk of cardiovascular disease the daily dosage of EPA and DHA combined should be at least 1,000 mg.

A MATTER OF PERSPECTIVE . . .

The next issue I want to address is the perception many people have that drugs are safe but dietary supplements are dangerous. It amazes me that adverse reactions to prescription drugs are estimated to kill more than 100,000 Americans every year, yet the media seem to be interested only in inaccurately portraying the dietary supplement industry as dangerous and "unregulated." I think a better perspective is in order. I agree that some natural products pose health risks and are potentially harmful, but on the whole there is significantly greater risk with many over-the-counter and prescription drugs. Even a drug as casually used as aspirin can produce serious side effects; it is a well-established fact that each year aspirin and other NSAIDs (nonsteroidal anti-inflammatory drugs) account for an estimated 16,500 deaths and 100,000 hospitalizations in the United States. The NSAIDs include aspirin, ibuprofen, naproxen, diclofenac, ketoprofen, and tiaprofenic acid as well as the new, much maligned COX-2 inhibitors such as Vioxx and Celebrex.

Even though less than 10 percent of all adverse drug reactions (ADRs) are ever reported to the FDA with regard to prescription and over-the-counter drugs, the data that do exist on the scope of the problem are sobering. For example, on the basis of detailed analysis and projections presented in the most respected medical journals, including the *Journal of the American*

Medical Association, it is estimated that 6.7 percent of hospitalized patients have a serious ADR, with a fatality rate of 0.32 percent. This translates to more than 2.2 million serious ADRs in hospitalized patients, causing more than 106,000 deaths annually. These statistics do not include ADRs that occur outside hospitals, or the estimated 350,000 ADRs that occur in U.S. nursing homes each year. Moreover, as noted above ADRs are substantially underreported.[9, 10, 11]

If we use these statistics to calculate monetary figures, the cost of drug-related illness and mortality is probably now more than $200 billion annually. To put this dollar amount into perspective, it is more than the total cost of treating diabetes or heart disease in the United States. The obvious question is, "Why are there so many ADRs?" There are many reasons. Here are just a few.

- First, more people are being placed on drugs now than ever before. For example, about 5 billion prescriptions were filled last year. That is about 12 prescriptions for every person in the United States.

- Second, more and more people are being placed on combinations of drugs—often because additional drugs are needed to deal with side effects caused by the original drugs. The rate of ADRs increases exponentially after a patient is on four or more medications.

- Third, many of the newer drugs are more dangerous than older drugs. The FDA has approved many of these new drugs without having complete data on their safety. Drug companies can now pay a fee to speed up approval. Of the 548 new drugs approved by the FDA from 1975 to 1999, 56 (10 percent) were given a new "Black Box Warning" because of severe ADRs or were withdrawn from the market because of reports of deaths.

- Fourth, the majority of complaints for which patients see doctors originate in dietary and lifestyle factors. Trying to treat the symptoms with a drug (a biochemical Band-Aid) fails to address the underlying cause, and the drug itself leads to side effects.

MISGUIDED CONCERN

Recently, *Consumer Reports* came up with what it referred to as the "dirty dozen" among natural products. When you take a look at the list as a whole, it is laughable that these were presented as a public health concern, both because of what is listed and because the risk is insignificant compared with ADRs.

Consumer Reports' Dirty Dozen

Androstenedione (andro, for short)

Aristolochic acid

Bitter orange

Chaparral

Comfrey

Germander

Kava (or kava kava)

Lobelia

Organ and glandular extracts

Pennyroyal oil

Skullcap

Yohimbe

I agree that androstenedione (andro) is certainly not a dietary supplement and that aristolochic acid and pennyroyal oil are definitely hazardous, but most of the health food stores that I have been in do not carry these products or others on the list. For example, the natural product industry has been aware of the dangers of comfrey root's pyrrolizidine alkaloids for more than 20 years. In fact, I haven't seen a comfrey root product designed for oral use containing these compounds in a health food store in the last twenty years or so. I could be wrong—there could be some comfrey out there being sold as a tea. But my point is that comfrey is really not a public health hazard. If you take a good look at some of the other members of the "dirty dozen," you will see that they pose little risk simply because they are not widely available. How many people in the last decade have had an adverse reaction to comfrey or the others?

The media keep harping on the dangers of ephedra, a source of the stimulant ephedrine that was used in combination with caffeine to aid weight loss. But was ephedra really all that bad? My feeling is that the abuse of ephedra was the primary issue. If ephedra is used responsibly at appropriate dosages, there is no question that it is a safe and effective natural product. Granted, there was a tendency toward abuse, because Americans typically believe that if a little is good, a lot is even better. But again, let's try to keep things in perspective. In the worst case scenario, over the last 20 years ephedra was linked to approximately 150 deaths (virtually all of which were related to excessive dosage or abuse). In contrast, there were approximately 2 million deaths in the United States from ADRs, including more than 140,000 deaths caused by aspirin and other NSAIDs.

Taking anything by mouth—whether it is a food, a drug, or a supplement—requires some personal responsibility. But the relative risk of danger from taking a nutritional supplement or herbal product is substantially less than that seen with prescription and over-the-counter drugs. This fact is very clear.

A DIETARY SUPPLEMENT PRIMER

What distinguishes a dietary supplement such as a vitamin, mineral, or herbal product from a drug is that a dietary supplement must not claim to treat, cure, or prevent disease even if it obviously does have such effects. A product sold as a dietary supplement and touted on its labeling as a new treatment or cure for a specific disease or condition would be considered an unapproved—and thus illegal—drug. The FDA allows manufacturers of supplements to refer to a supplement's effect on bodily structure or function, including its overall effect on a person's well-being. Such references are known as structure-function claims. Examples of structure-function claims are:

- ▸ Calcium builds strong bones.

- ▸ Antioxidants maintain cell integrity.

- ▸ Fiber maintains bowel regularity.

As with any food product, federal law requires manufacturers of dietary supplements to ensure that the products they put on the market are safe. It is the FDA's responsibility to police the safety of nutritional supplements. The FDA must show that a dietary supplement is unsafe before it can take action to restrict the product's use or take the product off the market. The Dietary Supplement and Nonprescription Drug Consumer Protection Act of 1994 was designed to increase reporting of serious side effects from dietary supplements. Labels will have to feature a U.S. address or phone number to which reports of serious adverse events can be directed. I am confident that even with this new regulation, dietary supplements will continue to have a tremendous reputation for safety.

WHY IS THERE SUCH A BIAS?

In 1998, an article in *Archives of Internal Medicine* by James Goodwin M.D. and Michael Tangum M.D. highlighted what most physicians who prescribe nutritional supplements as medicines have been saying for years: there is a clear bias in conventional medical circles against nutritional supplementation.[12] Medical bias, regardless of type, represents an abandonment of scientific impartiality and of the search for truth. The bias results largely because doctors, researchers, medical colleges, drug companies, and other vested interests want to maintain the status quo. Professional self-interest and profit are regarded as being more important than integrity and the best interests of patients.

As Dr. Goodwin and Dr. Tangum pointed out, the bias against and re-

Tips for Buying Supplements

Obviously, the current situation regarding the regulation, label claims, and intended use of natural products is less than ideal. As a person who has dedicated his life to understanding how these products work, and who is closely involved in the natural product industry, I know firsthand the relative merits of particular natural products. There is a tremendous gap between the purposes for which these products can be used safely and effectively and what the manufacturer is allowed to tell consumers. In addition, it is unfortunate that many products on the market provide little benefit, despite overstated claims.

I am a strong advocate of responsible self-care with natural products because I know that they can make a huge difference in the quality of life. However, I am also aware that many products on the market do not fulfill label claims and are of extremely poor quality. Though in most situations I cannot tell you exactly what product or brand to buy, I can offer you some general guidance. My most important recommendation is to buy from respected manufacturers within the health food industry that follow good manufacturing practice (GMP). A manufacturer that follows the FDA's guidelines for GMP is the most likely to have a high-quality product. Here is a practical tip: if the price of one product is substantially less than that of a seemingly identical product, buy the more expensive one. With nutritional and herbal products (like many other things), you get what you pay for. A company that follows appropriate GMP and has its own quality-control laboratory will have a higher overhead then a manufacturer who does not follow GMP and as a result will have to charge more for its product.

sistance to nutritional interventions are evidenced in at least three ways: (1) uncritical acceptance of any news pertaining to toxicity, (2) use of an angry and scornful tone in discussions of nutritional supplementation in the leading textbooks of medicine, and (3) ignoring of evidence supporting the benefits or therapeutic efficacy of nutritional supplements.

The example used in the article to support the first point is the uncritical acceptance of the notion that vitamin C (ascorbic acid) can cause oxalate kidney stones. This unsubstantiated, long-standing opinion is written as law in most medical textbooks. But there are no data to support it. Administration of up to 10 grams (g) per day of vitamin C has not shown any effect on urinary oxalate. In the large-scale Harvard Prospective Health Professional Follow-Up Study, those groups in the highest quintile of vitamin C intake (> 1500 mg/day) had a lower risk of kidney stones than the groups in the lowest quintiles. Despite this evidence, the myth that vitamin C causes kidney stones continues to be uncritically accepted and promulgated in major textbooks and review articles.

The examples provided for the second point—the angry and scornful tone adopted in discussions of nutritional supplementation in the leading textbooks of medicine—are numerous direct quotations from several editions of two major American textbooks: Harrison's *Principles of Internal Medicine* and Cecil's *A Textbook of Medicine*. The words used include "false," "indefensible," "wasteful," "unnecessary," "deplored," and "poor medical practice."

The third point—ignoring evidence of benefit or therapeutic efficacy—is the most serious problem because it has the effect of withholding potentially life-changing and even lifesaving therapies. The example used in the article is that despite numerous controlled clinical trials demonstrating that in the treatment of intermittent claudication vitamin E is at least as effective as vasodilators (but without side effects), no mention is made of this fact in any of the thirteen editions of Cecil's *A Textbook of Medicine* or the twelve editions of Harrison's *Principles of Internal Medicine*. Although there are even better examples, it is surely a sign of bias that vitamin E has shown such good effects in improving intermittent claudication as well as decreasing the rate of leg amputation and overall mortality but is not even mentioned in any of these editions.

Why the resistance? For some reason, resistance to nutritional science has been deeply ingrained for more than 200 years. Keep in mind that the medical community and the British navy did not give a ration of lime juice to naval crews until 1804, 62 years after the discovery and proof offered by the British physician James Lind in 1742 that lime juice prevents scurvy. The process seems to run a little faster now, but it is still too slow for the adoption of scientific information on the importance of nutrition into mainstream medical thought.

THE UNNECESSARY TIME LAG

In our current medical system there appears to be an unnecessary lag between the time when a vitamin or mineral is proved to be effective for preventing or treating a certain health condition and the time it becomes widely accepted and is recommended by physicians. A case in point is the time lag between the demonstration and the acceptance of the role folic acid plays in the prevention of neural-tube defects such as spina bifida, a defect in which the vertebrae do not form a complete ring to protect the spinal cord.

The discovery that folic acid supplementation (400 mg per day) in early pregnancy can reduce the incidence of neural-tube defects by as much as 80 percent is regarded as one of the greatest findings of the last part of the twentieth century.[13] The evidence became so overwhelming that the FDA finally had to reverse its previous position and acknowledge the association, allowing folic acid supplements and foods high in folic acid to claim that "daily consumption of folic acid by women of childbearing age may reduce the risk of neural-tube defects."

The interesting thing concerning the discovery of the link between folic acid deficiency and neural-tube defects is how long it took for obstetricians and other medical doctors to begin making the recommendation of folic acid supplementation to pregnant women. In addition, given the safety of folic acid, why was the FDA so dead set against the possibility that it might help prevent such a serious birth defect? My feeling is that its attitude, again, was related to an inherent bias. That bias is getting in the way of the advancement of medicine and the health of Americans.

Once it became "accepted medical practice" to recommend folic acid to women of childbearing age, obstetricians felt they had to do everything possible to make sure their patients were taking folic acid, presumably to prevent a malpractice suit if a child was born with a neural-tube defect.

Although obstetricians and other medical doctors claim that the protective effects of folic acid were not known until 1992, when the U.S. Public Health Service issued a recommendation that all women of childbearing age capable of becoming pregnant should consume 400 mg of folic acid per day, folic acid deficiency was linked to neural-tube defects since the early 1960s. How long will it take the medical profession to accept other links related to nutritional supplementation in the treatment and prevention of disease?

There are countless examples of how supplementing one's diet with an inexpensive vitamin or mineral can have significant preventive or therapeutic effects, yet many physicians place an unnecessary burden of proof on the vitamin or mineral before they feel inclined to make such a recommendation. My message to these physicians is to rethink their position. Instead of waiting for absolute proof, they should ask whether there is reasonable certainty that a particular recommendation may be beneficial. What do I mean by "reasonable certainty"? Basically, does the recommendation make sense? Is there a good chance that the recommendation may be of value? Does it provide a favorable cost-to-benefit ratio? Is the recommendation safe?

MAGNESIUM SUPPLEMENTATION IN DIABETES

One of the best examples of a situation when the medical community has hesitated to recommend a nutritional supplement that would significantly reduce suffering and death is the use of magnesium supplements for diabetes. I am offering it here as a model nutritional recommendation that should be mainstream, as there is considerable evidence that diabetics should take supplemental magnesium.[14, 15, 16] The reasons: over half of all people with diabetes show evidence of magnesium deficiency; magnesium improves blood sugar control; and magnesium may prevent some of the complications of diabetes, such as retinopathy (eye disease) and heart disease. Magnesium is a mineral that resides primarily within the cells of the body, not the blood. When the blood level of magnesium is low, it means that the level in the cells is very low. Even when blood (serum) magnesium is used to assess status, levels are usually low in diabetics and lowest in those with diabetic complications such as retinopathy and neuropathy. Clinical studies have shown that magnesium supplementation (usually 400 to 500 mg per day) improves insulin response and action, blood sugar control, and the fluidity of red blood cells, enabling these cells to deliver oxygen better.

To deal with the growing evidence that magnesium supplementation is beneficial in the treatment of diabetes, the American Diabetes Association sponsored a consensus panel to examine the data and make a recommendation to physicians. This presumably expert panel clearly acknowledged the weight of the scientific literature supporting magnesium supplementation in diabetics and noted that serum (blood) magnesium does not reflect body magnesium stores, yet it cannot seem to realize that magnesium supplementation is appropriate for diabetics. In fact, "the panel recommends that patients with diabetes at increased risk of magnesium deficiency, but in whom such deficiencies cannot be demonstrated by clinically available tests, not receive magnesium supplementation." They believe that "adequate" dietary magnesium intake can generally be achieved by a nutritionally balanced meal plan as recommended by the American Diabetes Association.

This position strikes me as illogical. What the panel appears to be saying is something like, "Yes, we know that magnesium is critical to the regulation of blood glucose and blood pressure, as well as for the possible prevention of complications of diabetes. We also know that magnesium supplementation has been shown to be beneficial in the treatment of diabetes and may enhance insulin sensitivity. We understand that current tests of magnesium status are not reflective of magnesium tissue stores. Yet despite all this information we cannot recommend magnesium supplementation unless a person has magnesium deficiency documented by a test (serum magnesium or urine magnesium) that reflects only 0.3 percent of the total body magnesium pool and is reduced only when the level of magnesium within cells is severely depleted."

The reason for the apparent contradiction is that this was a "consensus" panel. Even after Columbus returned from America, there were still those who argued that the world was flat. If a group of geographical experts in 1492 had been asked to make a consensus statement on the shape of the world, their conclusion would probably have sounded similar.

FINAL COMMENTS

One of the myths about nutritional supplementation has been that there is no firm scientific evidence to support it. However, this argument is quickly becoming outdated. There is more than enough reasonable certainty to use nutritional supplementation for virtually every common health condition. Yet nutritional supplementation is still an undervalued and underused therapy because of selective bias in conventional medical circles. To borrow from closing comments by James Goodwin, and Michael Tangum, in their editorial on bias against nutritional supplementation, the merits of nutritional supplementation should be based on its benefits versus its risks, safety, and cost. They write: "Issues such as the theory underlying the treatment or the guild to which the proponents of the treatment belong should be irrelevant." Eventually this enlightened thinking will prevail and conventional medicine will embrace nutritional supplementation as a preventive and therapeutic measure.

11

HOW TO GET WELL

*"Nature is doing her best each moment to make us well.
She exists for no other end. Do not resist. With the
least inclination to be well, we should not be sick."*
—Henry David Thoreau

WE LIVE IN A society where there is tremendous confusion about the concept of wellness and health. I am of the belief that health and wellness are much more than merely the absence of disease or illness. I am not alone in this belief. The World Health Organization (WHO) defines health as "a state of complete physical, mental, and social well being, not merely the absence of disease or infirmity." This definition provides a positive range of health well beyond the absence of sickness. The difference between wellness and health is that the term "wellness" also includes emotional and spiritual aspects of life.

To achieve wellness involves a systems approach. This means that attention has to be given to all areas, as every component of our life affects another. Wellness requires a "whole person" perspective that includes the myriad of choices we make—our attitudes, habits, diet, lifestyle, etc. You absolutely must realize that getting well is achieved by taking personal responsibility for your life, your current situation, and your health; and that every aspect of your life must be utilized to propel you toward the goal of wellness. The question of health or disease often comes down to individual responsibility. In this context, responsibility means choosing a healthy alternative over a less healthy one. If you want to be healthy, simply make healthy choices on a consistent basis.

No matter what your current state of wellness might be, you can take steps to improve it. Keep in mind that the human body is constantly regenerating itself. For example, every three to four days we have a whole new lining in the gastrointestinal tract as new cells are formed to replace damaged old cells. In just 30 days, we renew our entire skin. Every six weeks, we make an entirely new liver. We live within a vessel of incredible complexity adapted to propel us through life. Though we might abuse it for a while, our body is very forgiving if we give it the right support and enough time.

IT'S CRAZY NOT TO BE A HEALTH NUT

My new patient, Anne, was dealing with health issues typical of a 65-year-old woman living in the United States—osteoporosis, high cholesterol, high blood pressure, arthritis, ulcers, and diabetes. When I met her in the lobby of our clinic, I was enthusiastically greeted by her sister, Elizabeth—a vibrant, healthy-looking, attractive middle-aged woman. I later learned from Anne that her being in my office was all Elizabeth's doing. Anne went on to tell me that all her siblings—two brothers and two other sisters—were fighting the same sort of ailments that she was, except for her "younger" sister, Elizabeth. When I said that perhaps Elizabeth would fall prey to the same fate, she just smiled and said, "I don't think so." I was a bit curious about her inflection of "younger" and her obvious disapproval regarding something about her sister, so I asked her how much younger Elizabeth was. Well, Anne told me that Elizabeth was actually 8 years older than herself, and the oldest sibling in the family. I was shocked because whereas Anne looked closer to 80 than to 65, Elizabeth looked like a woman in her mid-fifties. I could not resist—I asked Anne why she felt Elizabeth would be spared the diseases that were afflicting the other members of the family. Her response was stated with distain, "Oh, she has been a health nut for fifty years." At that moment I truly realized how absolutely insane it is for anyone not to be a health nut. We are given one body to nourish and serve us. Why not make it as healthy as possible?

I felt that Anne, like many patients who are more or less coerced by a family member into seeing me, might not be receptive to the dietary, lifestyle, and supplementation strategies that I would lay out to address her health issues. She belonged to an era that for some reason rejected the notion of diet and lifestyle as fundamental to healing. Instead, she chose to rely on "a few little pills"—actually, she was on 11 different medications—to try to correct her faulty biochemistry. Experience had taught me the best way to handle such a situation. I simply asked Anne if she was willing to make any changes to her diet and lifestyle. When she said no, I quickly but graciously ended the appointment. Since we had only used 15 of the allotted 45 minutes, I had an opportunity to spend some time with Elizabeth. It was inspiring to me to see so vividly how following a path of health could help someone defy the odds of developing heritable diseases and could dramatically slow down the aging process.

For nearly 30 years I have lived the life of a health nut—so I have not only talked the talk; I have walked the walk and helped others do the same. Over this time, I have been interested to see many components of the natural health movement in the 1970s and 1980s become part of the mainstream—yogurt, salad bars, whole grains, vitamin and mineral supplements, tofu, soy milk, etc. But for some illogical reason a stigma still remains: if you care about your body and health, you are "nuts." There also seems to be in society a deep underlying tendency to reject the idea that diet, lifestyle, and natural medicines offer an effective answer to the health challenges facing America, even though there is tremendous support for this idea.

In our information age, most people know what they need to do to be healthy, live longer, lose weight, etc. The disconnect is between that knowledge and the effective execution of the strategy. In this chapter I will detail the necessary steps to wellness, but you and you alone will have to take those steps.

THE SEVEN STEPS TO WELLNESS

The title of this chapter pays homage to *How to Get Well*, by Paavo Airola, published in 1974. It was one of the first books I read when I started making choices to achieve wellness in my own life. Paavo Airola was one of the premier natural health educators of the 1970s and, along with Adele Davis, was responsible for creating much of the initial momentum of the natural health movement. I have learned a lot since I read Airola's landmark book. My goal in this chapter is to summarize the salient points from his book, from my own experience with patients, and from other books as clear-cut, easy-to-follow steps to wellness.

- Step 1—Incorporate spirituality in your life.

- Step 2—Develop a positive mental attitude.

- Step 3—Focus on establishing positive relationships.

- Step 4—Follow a healthy lifestyle.

- Step 5—Be active and get regular physical exercise.

- Step 6—Eat a health-promoting diet.

- Step 7—Support your body through proper nutritional supplementation and body work.

STEP 1—INCORPORATE
SPIRITUALITY IN YOUR LIFE

Spirituality means different things to different people. For me, it means recognizing that there is a power greater than myself, which connects us all. I know that many people try to get through life without faith, religion, or God, but quite frankly I don't see how life could have much meaning without them. And I believe that incorporating spirituality in our lives can have a profound effect on our health—however or whatever you imagine God to be.

In Chapter 2, I highlighted the importance of some aspects of spirituality in healing. As a physician, I have reached the conclusion that the most powerful medicine of all may have nothing to do with drugs, surgery, or other medical "magic bullets." I have seen firsthand that the human spirit is a source of phenomenal healing and can create miracles when science falls short. In order to incorporate more spirituality in your life, I believe that you must focus on seven "keys":

- ► Key 1. Realize the power of prayer. Prayer elicits the relaxation response, promotes healing, and connects us to our inner self and God.

- ► Key 2. Make prayer part of your daily routine. Set aside time in your day, every day, to acknowledge the good in your life and be thankful. Bless those you care about and ask for guidance for those you don't.

- ► Key 3. Read a spiritual guide (e.g., the Bible or the Koran) or some other inspirational book on a daily basis. Recognize that we all need to be reminded of our true path in life. We require guidelines and inspiration to stay the course.

- ► Key 4. Use the power of love. It is true that love heals all. Before we can love others, we must first learn to love and accept ourselves so that we can become more accepting and loving of others.

- ► Key 5. Create a vehicle in your life that makes a difference in the life of others. Giving is part of our nature, and we must have a vehicle through which to express it. Making a difference in life does not have to be anything on a grand scale. The biggest impact that most of us will have is on those around us whom we care about, particularly our family.

- ► Key 6. Tithe or give to charity. Giving, in a material sense, is a sign of our commitment to trying to make the world a better place.

- ► Key 7. Reinforce your faith. Spending time with others of like mind, whether attending a church or not, allows for expression of your spirituality and the ability to extend love to others.

STEP 2—DEVELOP A POSITIVE
MENTAL ATTITUDE

The importance of a positive mental attitude was discussed briefly in Chapter 8. As I have seen over and over in my patients' lives (and my own life), it is not what happens to us that determines our direction; rather, our response to those challenges shapes the quality of our life and determines to a very large degree our level of health. Surprisingly, hardship, heartbreak, disappointment, and failure often serve as the spark for joy, ecstasy, compassion, and success. The determining factor is whether we view these challenges as stumbling blocks or stepping-stones. Optimism is not only a necessary step toward achieving optimal health; it is critical to happiness and a higher quality of life.

Detailed evidence supports the contention that optimists live longer, suffer from fewer and less severe diseases (including cancer), and are much healthier than pessimists. During a 30-year study conducted by researchers at the prestigious Mayo Clinic in Rochester, Minnesota, the survival rate of optimists was 19 percent greater than that of pessimists.[1] What this number means is that 19 percent fewer optimists died during the study, as compared with pessimists. All causes of death were reduced in optimists, including cancer.

Here are the keys for step 2.

▸ Key 1. Become an optimist. The term "optimism" comes from the Latin *optimum*, meaning "the greatest good." Optimism is the philosophy that looks for the best possible outcome and that focuses on the most hopeful aspects of a situation. To test your level of optimism, see Appendix A (pages 263–273).

▸ Key 2. Practice positive self-talk. We all conduct a continual running dialogue in our heads. In time, what we say to ourselves will percolate down into our subconscious mind. Those thoughts, in turn, affect the way we think and feel. Naturally, if you feed yourself a steady stream of negative thoughts—"I'm no good; I hate myself; I hate the world"—your subconscious will respond in kind. Become aware of your self-talk, and then consciously work to feed positive messages to your subconscious mind.

▸ Key 3. Ask better questions. The quality of your life is equal to the quality of the questions you habitually ask yourself. For example, if you experience a setback, do you think, "Why am I so stupid? Why do bad things always happen to me?" Or do you think, "OK, what can I learn from this so that it never happens again? What can I do to make the situation better?" Clearly, the latter response is healthier. Regardless of the specific situation, asking better questions is bound to improve your attitude.

▸ Key 4. Use affirmations. An affirmation is a positive statement with some emotional intensity behind it. Affirmations can make an imprint on the subconscious mind to create a healthy, positive self-image. In addition, affirmations can actually fuel the changes you desire. I use certain phrases and sentences as affirmations each day. I have these affirmations in plain sight on my desk:

  ▷ I am blessed with an abundance of energy!

  ▷ Love, joy, and happiness flow through me with every heartbeat.

  ▷ I am thankful to God for all my good fortune!

  ▷ YES I CAN!

▸ Key 5. Set positive goals. Learning to set achievable goals is a powerful method for building a positive attitude and raising self-esteem. Achieving goals creates a success cycle: you feel better about yourself; and the better you feel about yourself, the more likely you are to succeed. Here are some guidelines for setting health goals:

  ▷ State the goal in positive terms and in the present tense; avoid negative words. Don't say, "I will not eat sugar, candy, ice cream, and other fattening foods." It's better to say, "I enjoy eating healthy, low-calorie, nutritious foods."

▷ Make your goal attainable and realistic. Start out with goals that are easily attainable, like drinking six glasses of water a day and switching from white bread to whole wheat. By initially choosing easily attainable goals, you create a success cycle that helps build a positive self-image. Little things add up to make a major difference in the way you feel about yourself.

▷ Be specific. The more clearly you define your goal, the more likely you are to reach it. For example, if you want to lose weight, what is the weight you desire? What body fat percentage or measurements do you want to achieve?

▸ Key 6. Use positive visualizations. Imagery is another powerful tool in achieving health, happiness, or success. I believe that we have to be able to see our life as we want it to be before it happens. With regard to health, you absolutely must picture yourself in ideal health if you truly want to experience this state. Our dreams propel us as we roll through life. They are powerful and inspirational.

▸ Key 7. Read or listen to positive messages. Again, we all need to be reminded of our true path in life. We require guidelines and inspiration to stay the course.

STEP 3—FOCUS ON ESTABLISHING POSITIVE RELATIONSHIPS

Human beings need one another. We need relationships. We need to work with others, exchange services, share information, and provide emotional comfort. Positive human relationships sustain us and nourish us—in body and soul. There is much scientific evidence that positive relationships can prevent disease and extend life. Conversely, negative close relationships or a lack of close confidants can be very harmful to our health. A poor marital relationship is linked to heart attacks, heart failure, metabolic syndrome, and type 2 diabetes. In one very detailed study, British civil servants filled out a questionnaire that assessed their relationship status.[2] Of 8,499 individuals who did not have coronary heart disease (CHD) at the beginning of the study and who provided sufficient information for analysis, 589 reported a CHD event (e.g., heart attack). After adjusting for variables such as obesity, hypertension, diabetes, cholesterol, smoking, alcohol intake, exercise, and consumption of fruits and vegetables, the researchers found that people who experienced negative aspects of a close relationship had a 34 percent higher risk of coronary events than those who did not. The researchers concluded that to avoid CHD and live longer people needed to "be nicer to each other." Here are the keys for positive relationships.

▶ Key 1. Learn to listen. The quality of any relationship ultimately comes down to the quality of communication. The biggest roadblock to effective communication in most relationships is poor listening skills. When we are truly listening, we are telling the other person that he or she is important to us and that we respect and love him or her. In other words, listening is an active demonstration of love and respect in our relationships. Here are seven tips to good listening that I found easy to learn and quite useful. (Some of these were introduced in Chapter 3.)

▷ Tip 1. Do not interrupt. Allow the people you are communicating with to share their feelings and thoughts uninterrupted. Empathize with them; put yourself in their shoes. If you first seek to understand, you will find yourself being better understood.

▷ Tip 2. Be an active listener. This means that you must act really interested in what other people are communicating. Listen to what they are saying instead of thinking about your response. Ask questions to gain more information or clarify what they are telling you. Good questions open lines of communication.

▷ Tip 3. Be a reflective listener. Restate or reflect back to others your interpretation of what they are telling you. This simple technique shows them that you are both listening to and understanding what they are saying. Restating what you think is being said may cause short-term conflict in some situations, but it is certainly worth the risk. Just explain that you want to be certain you understand what others are trying to say.

▷ Tip 4. Wait to speak until the people you want to communicate with are listening. If they are not ready to listen, no matter how well you communicate, your message will not be heard.

▷ Tip 5. Don't try to talk over somebody. If you find yourself being interrupted, relax. Don't try to outtalk the other person. If you are courteous and allow others to speak, eventually (unless they are extremely rude), they will respond likewise. If they don't point out that they are interrupting the communication process. You can do this only if you yourself have been a good listener. Double standards in relationships seldom work.

▷ Tip 6. Help others become active listeners. Ask them if they understood what you were communicating. Ask them to tell you what they heard. If they don't seem to understand what you are saying, keep explaining until they do.

▷ Tip 7. Don't be afraid of long silences. Human communication involves much more than words. Unfortunately, in many situations silence can make us feel uncomfortable, but a great deal can be communicated during silences. Relax. Some people need silence to collect their thoughts and feel safe in communicating. The important thing to remember during silences is that you must remain an active listener.

▶ Key 2. Develop positive personal values. Our values define who we really are. Values are learned, so we can change our lives by changing our values. Values ultimately allow us to receive love and acceptance from our friends and family. Develop positive values and you will be blessed with very gratifying and rewarding relationships. Here are some universal positive values that are respected by all:

▷ Honesty

▷ Loyalty

▷ Integrity

▷ Sincerity

▷ Humility

▷ Enthusiasm

▷ Dedication

▷ Dependability

▷ A sense of humor

▷ Open-mindedness

▸ Key 3. Learn to help others. Our nature is to be giving, to be altruistic, to have an unselfish concern for the welfare of others. Although its focus is on others, altruism serves us indirectly. To illustrate this point, here is a favorite story of mine from Zig Zigler's book *See You at the Top*:

> A man was given a tour of both Heaven and Hell, so he could intelligently select his final destination. The Devil was given first chance, so he started the "prospect" with a tour of Hell. The first glance was a surprising one because all occupants were seated at a banquet table loaded with every food imaginable, including meat from every corner of the globe, fruits and vegetables and every delicacy known to man. With justification, the Devil pointed out that no one could ask for more.
>
> However, when the man looked carefully at the people he did not find a single smile. He heard no music nor did he see any indication of the gaiety generally associated with such a feast. The people at the table looked dull and listless and were literally skin and bones. The tourist noticed that each person had a fork strapped to the left arm and a knife strapped to the right arm. Each had a four

foot handle which made it impossible to eat. So, with food of every kind at their fingertips, they were starving.

Next stop was Heaven, where the tourist saw a scene identical in every respect—same foods, knives and forks with those four-foot handles. However, the inhabitants of Heaven were laughing, singing, and having a great time. They were well fed and in excellent health. The tourist was puzzled for a moment. He wondered how conditions could be so similar and yet produce such different results. The people in Hell were starving and miserable, while the people in heaven were well-fed and happy. Then, he saw the reason. Each person in Hell had been trying to feed himself. A knife and fork with a four-foot handle made this impossible. Each person in Heaven was feeding the one across the table from him and was being fed by the one sitting on the opposite side. By helping one another, they helped themselves.

▸ Key 4. Find and look for the good in others. The way that you see others has an effect on how you relate to them, how they view you, and how you view yourself. If you constantly criticize and look for negative traits in people, this attitude will be reflected back to you. If we can focus our attention on the positive, if we can look for the good in people and situations, that becomes more of our reality. To be happy and have positive relationships, you absolutely must become a good finder. You must look for the good in people. You must expect the best from people. And you must reinforce the good that you see.

▸ Key 5. Demonstrate love and appreciation. It is not enough to simply feel love in our friendships and intimate relationships; we must express these feelings. We must demonstrate to our loved ones just how important they are to us. We must continually find ways to communicate our deepest feelings through our actions, whether orally, in writing, through touch, or by our behavior. We all need to see, hear, and physically feel love and appreciation.

▸ Key 6. Develop intimacy. Intimacy is very important to good health. It probably relates to the nurturing that takes place when we share our deepest selves. Intimate relationships are the most gratifying. However, many people have a hard time developing a truly intimate relationship—especially with their spouse. Here is a simple tip that I have found to help nourish intimacy. Take a walk together. Moving together physically really opens up communication. It has to do with body language and a phenomenon called "mirroring and matching." Adopting another person's speech, body language, or behavior triggers our subconscious to develop a feeling of rapport. The next time you are in a restaurant, take a look around and notice how many people (especially lovers) are mirroring and matching. You'll be amazed. Try using mirroring and matching to your advantage to enhance intimacy. It is very powerful. If you have few intimate relationships in your life, you need to reach out and establish more friendships. Here are three additional tips you may find useful.

▷ Attend workshops, seminars, and classes you are interested in. You will find people who share your beliefs and interests—fertile ground for developing supportive friendships.

▷ Become a volunteer at a local hospital, a school, a nursing home, or any other place where you can really make a difference.

▷ Get a pet. A relationship with a pet can be almost as positive as human relationship. Studies have shown that owning or caring for a pet can relieve loneliness, depression, and anxiety, and even promote a quicker recovery from illness.

▸ Key 7. Recognize challenges in relationships and be courageous in dealing with them. Even the best relationships experience stress. In fact, these "stress points" actually strengthen a relationship. This is particularly true in marriages.

STEP 4—FOLLOW A HEALTHY LIFESTYLE

Our lifestyle reflects our daily habits. In many ways, these habits define our health. By avoiding harmful habits and embracing health-promoting habits we can transform our lives toward wellness. Here are the seven keys to a healthy lifestyle. (Note: Exercise is so important it is dealt with separately.)

▸ Key 1. Do not smoke. Smoking is still the most preventable cause of cancer and premature death in the United States. Smoking is associated with an increased risk of virtually every cancer (not just lung cancer) and accounts for at least 30 percent of all deaths from cancer. Smoking is also a major cause of heart disease (the leading cause of death in the United States), strokes, chronic bronchitis, and emphysema. Here are 10 tips for stopping smoking:

1. List all the reasons why you want to quit smoking and review them daily.

2. Set a specific day to quit, tell at least 10 friends that you are going to quit smoking, and then *do it*!

3. Use substitutes. Instead of smoking, chew on raw vegetables, fruits, or gum. If your fingers seem empty, play with a pencil.

4. Avoid situations that you associate with smoking.

5. When you need to relax, perform deep breathing exercises rather than reaching for a cigarette.

6. Realize that 40 million Americans have quit. If they can do it, so can you!

7. Visualize yourself as a nonsmoker with more available money, pleasant breath, unstained teeth, and the satisfaction that comes from being in control of your life.

8. Join a support group. Call the local American Cancer Society and ask for referrals. You are not alone.

9. Each day, reward yourself in a positive way. Buy yourself something with the money you've saved, or plan a special reward as a celebration for quitting.

10. Take one day at a time.

► Key 2. Drink alcohol only in moderation. Alcohol is our nation's number one drug problem, as it seriously affects the health of more than 10 million people. Although moderate drinking (no more than one or two drinks per day) has actually been shown to be associated with a longer life, excessive drinking is strongly associated with five of the leading causes of death in the United States: accidents, cirrhosis of the liver, pneumonia, suicide, and murder.

► Key 3. Get adequate rest. Your body needs sleep to function properly. During sleep, the body repairs itself. Without sufficient sleep, needed repairs go undone, and the body is more likely to break down. Exactly how much sleep you need depends on you. Some people find that they need only five or six hours of sleep; others may need 10 or 11. Regardless of how much sleep you think you might require, the truth of the matter is that most Americans do not get enough sleep to function optimally. In addition, at least 40 million Americans suffer from insomnia or some other sleep disturbance. To improve your ability to sleep, see page 175 for seven tips.

► Key 4. Develop a positive way to manage stress. Let's face it: everyday stress is a normal part of modern living. Job pressures, family arguments, financial pressures, traffic, and time management are just a few of the stressors we face on a daily basis. Whether you are aware of it or not, you have developed a pattern for coping with stress. Unfortunately, most people have found patterns and methods that do not support good health. These include negative patterns such as overeating, uncontrolled emotional outbursts, feelings of helplessness, having a cocktail or beer, or smoking a cigarette. It is important for you to identify any negative pattern and replace it with positive ways of coping. I believe that effective stress management involves four equally important areas:

▷ Techniques to calm the mind (see page 35) and promote a positive mental attitude.

▷ Following a healthy lifestyle, including regular physical exercise.

  ▷ Eating a healthful diet.

  ▷ Utilizing key dietary and botanical supplements that can improve
    the ability to deal with stress.

▸ Key 5. Effective time management. One of the biggest sources of
  stress and frustration for most people is time. They simply do not feel
  they have enough of it. By the way, time management does not mean
  squeezing more and more work into less and less time. It means
  learning to plan your time more effectively so that you allow time for
  the activities you enjoy.

▸ Key 6. Connect with nature. Most Americans spend 90 percent of
  their lives indoors, separated from fresh air, natural sunlight, and
  nature. Something extremely refreshing and calming happens when
  we can get in touch with nature, whether we simply take walk
  through a park or get out in the wilderness for a weekend of
  camping.

▸ Key 7. Laugh long and often—laughter is without question the most
  powerful medicine available. Recent medical research has confirmed
  that laughter enhances the blood flow to the body's extremities, and
  improves cardiovascular function, plays an active part in the body's
  release of endorphins and other natural mood-elevating and
  painkilling chemicals, boosts the immune system, and improves the
  transfer of oxygen and nutrients to internal organs. Here are seven tips
  that will help you have more laughter in your life:

  ▷ Learn to laugh at yourself. Recognize how funny some of your
    behavior really is—especially your shortcomings or mistakes. We all
    have little idiosyncrasies or behaviors that are unique to us and that
    we can recognize and enjoy. Do not take yourself too seriously.

  ▷ Inject humor any time it is appropriate. People love to laugh. Get a
    joke book and learn how to tell a good joke. Humor and laughter
    really make life enjoyable.

▷ Read the comics, find one that you think is funny, and follow it every day or week.

▷ Watch comedies on television. With modern cable systems, it is usually quite easy to find something funny on television.

▷ Go to see a funny movie with a friend. We laugh harder and more often when we are around others who are laughing. Laughter is contagious; we feed off each other's laughter; and laughing together helps people build good relationships.

▷ Listen to comedy audiotapes in your car while driving. Check your local audio store, bookstore, video store, or library for recorded routines of your favorite comedian.

▷ Play with kids. Kids really know how to laugh and play. If you do not have kids of your own, spend time with nieces, nephews, or neighborhood children with whose families you are friendly. Become a Big Brother or Sister. Investigate local Little Leagues. Help out at your church's Sunday school and children's events.

STEP 5—BE ACTIVE AND GET REGULAR PHYSICAL EXERCISE

The immediate effect of exercise is stress on the body, but with regular exercise the body adapts; it becomes stronger, functions more efficiently, and has greater endurance. The entire body benefits from regular exercise, largely as a result of improved cardiovascular and respiratory function. Exercise enhances the transport of oxygen and nutrients into cells. At the same time, exercise enhances the transport of carbon dioxide and waste products from the tissues of the body to the bloodstream and then to the eliminative organs. As a result, regular exercise increases stamina and energy.

Regular exercise is also powerful prescription for a positive mood. Tension, depression, feelings of inadequacy, and worries diminish greatly with regular exercise. Exercise alone has been demonstrated to have a tremendous impact on improving mood and the ability to handle stressful life situations.

Benefits of Exercise

Musculoskeletal System

Increases muscle strength

Increases flexibility of muscles and range of joint motion

Produces stronger bones, ligaments, and tendons

Lessens chance of injury

Enhances posture, poise, and physique

Prevents osteoporosis

Heart and Blood Vessels

Lowers resting heart rate

Strengthens heart function

Lowers blood pressure

Improves oxygen delivery throughout the body

Increases blood supply to muscles

Enlarges the arteries to the heart

Reduces the risk of heart disease

Helps lower blood cholesterol and triglyceride levels

Raises levels of HDL, the "good" cholesterol

Other Bodily Processes

Improves immune function

Aids digestion and elimination

Increases endurance and energy

Promotes lean body mass; burns fat

Mental Processes

Provides a natural release for pent-up feelings

Helps reduce tension and anxiety

Improves mental outlook and self-esteem

Helps relieve moderate depression

Improves the ability to handle stress

Stimulates improved mental function

Induces relaxation and improves sleep

Increases self-esteem

Exercise promotes the development of an efficient method to burn fat. Muscle tissue is the primary user of fat calories in the body. So, the greater your muscle mass, the greater your capacity to burn fat. Physical inactivity is a major reason why so many Americans are overweight. If you want to be healthy and achieve your ideal body weight, you *must* exercise.

Here are seven keys for step 5.

▸ Key 1. Recognize the importance of physical exercise. The first key is realizing just how important it is to get regular exercise. Regular exercise is vital to your health, but this fact means nothing unless it really sinks in and you accept it. You must make regular exercise a top priority in your life.

▸ Key 2. Consult your physician. If you are not currently on a regular exercise program, if you have health problems, or if you are over 40 years of age, get medical clearance. The main concern is the functioning of your heart. Exercise can be quite harmful (and even fatal) if your heart is not able to meet the increased demands placed on it.

▸ Key 3. Select an activity you enjoy. If you are fit enough to begin, the next key is selecting an activity that you will enjoy. Using the list below, choose from one to five activities that you think you may enjoy—or add a choice or two of your own. Make a commitment to do one activity a day for at least 20 minutes, and preferably for an hour. Your goal should be to enjoy the activity. The important thing is to move your body enough to raise your pulse a bit above its resting rate.

  ▹ Bicycling

  ▹ Cross-country skiing

  ▹ Dancing

  ▹ Golfing

  ▹ Jazzercise

  ▹ Jogging

  ▹ Rollerblading

  ▹ Stationary bicycling

  ▹ Swimming

  ▹ Tennis

  ▹ Treadmill

  ▹ Walking

  ▹ Weight lifting

▸ Key 4. Monitor intensity. The intensity of exercise is determined by measuring your heart rate (the number of times your heart beats per minute). This determination can be made quickly by placing the index and middle finger of one hand on your opposite wrist, or on the side of your neck just below the angle of your jaw. Beginning with zero, count the number of heartbeats for six seconds. Simply add a zero to this number, and you have your pulse rate. For example, if you counted 14 beats, your heart rate would be 140. Would this be a good number? It depends on your "training zone." A quick and easy way to determine your maximum training heart rate is to subtract your age from 185. For example, if you are 40 years old your maximum heart rate would be 145. To determine the bottom of the training zone, subtract 20 from this number. In the case of a 40-year-old, this would be 125. So the training range for a 40-year-old would be between 125 and 145 beats per minute. For maximum health benefits, you must stay within your training zone or range and never exceed it.

► Key 5. Do it often. A minimum of 15 to 20 minutes of exercising at your training heart rate at least three times a week is necessary to gain any significant cardiovascular benefits from exercise. It is better to exercise at the lower end of your training zone for longer periods of time than it is to exercise at a higher intensity for shorter periods of time.

► Key 6. Exercise with others. To get the maximum benefit from exercise, make it enjoyable. One way to make it fun is to get a workout partner. For example, if you choose walking as your activity, here is a great way to make it fun: find one or two people in your neighborhood whom you would enjoy walking with. If you are meeting others, you will certainly be more regular than if you depend solely on your own intentions. Commit yourselves to walking three to five mornings or afternoons each week, and increase the duration from an initial 10 minutes to at least 30 minutes.

► Key 7. Stay motivated. No matter how committed you are to regular exercise, at some point in time you are going to be faced with a loss of enthusiasm for working out. Here is a suggestion: read or thumb through fitness magazines like *Shape, Men's Fitness,* and *Muscle and*

Fitness. Looking at pictures of people who are in great shape really inspires me. In addition, these magazines typically feature articles on new exercise routines that are fun and interesting.

STEP 6—EAT A HEALTH-PROMOTING DIET

Diet is fundamental to good health, yet few Americans spend much thought or time on designing a diet that will promote health. Far too many people have succumbed to the comforts of modern life: they are physically inactive and they rely on foods that provide temporary sensory gratification at the expense of true nourishment. As a result, there is an epidemic of diet-related disease in the United States. But, it's easy to give your body its best chance of maintaining or achieving health. The following are seven important keys to a health-promoting diet.

- ▸ Key 1. Eat to control blood sugar levels. Refined sugars, white flour products, and other sources of simple sugars are quickly absorbed into the bloodstream, causing a rapid rise in blood sugar that leads to poor blood sugar regulation, obesity, and eventually type 2 diabetes. The stress on the body that sugars cause, including secreting too much insulin, can also promote the growth of cancers and increase the risk of heart disease. So, we will make this simple recommendation: don't eat junk foods, and do pay attention to the glycemic impact of the food you eat. Two measures of glycemic impact are the glycemic index (GI) and glycemic load (GL). The GI refers to how quickly blood sugar levels will rise after you eat a certain amount of food; this index is based on a referenced amount of carbohydrate. However, since it doesn't tell you how much carbohydrate is in a typical serving of a particular food, another tool is also needed: the GL. This is a relatively new way to assess the impact of carbohydrates. It takes the GI into account but gives a more complete picture of the effect that a food has on blood sugar levels. The GL is based on how much carbohydrate you actually eat in a serving. A GL of 20 or more is high, a GL of 11 to 19 inclusive is medium, and a GL of 10 or less is low. For example, let's take a look at beets—a food with a high GL but a low GL. Although the carbohydrate in beetroot has a high GI, there isn't a lot of it, so a typical serving of cooked beetroot has a glycemic load that is relatively low, about 5. Thus, as long you eat a reasonable portion of food that has a low GL, the impact on blood sugar is acceptable, even if the food has a high GI. I recommend consuming no more than a GL of 20 for any three-hour period. Appendix E provides a list of GI, fiber content, and GL load of common foods.

▶ Key 2. Daily, eat five or more servings of vegetables and two servings of fruit. A diet rich in fruits and vegetables is your best bet for preventing virtually every chronic disease. This fact has been established time and again in scientific studies of large numbers of people. The evidence in support of this recommendation is so strong that it has been endorsed by U.S. government health agencies and by virtually every major medical organization, including the American Cancer Society. In particular, by selecting fruits and vegetables in a variety of colors—including red, orange, yellow, green, blue, and purple—you'll be giving your body the full spectrum of pigments with powerful antioxidant effects, as well as the nutrients it needs for optimal function and protection against disease. Here are some easy tips for increasing your consumption of vegetables and fruit:

▷ Buy many kinds of fruits and vegetables when you shop, so that you have plenty of choices.

▷ Stock up on frozen vegetables so that you can have a vegetable dish with every dinner. You can easily steam frozen vegetables.

▷ Use the fruits and vegetables that go bad quickly, such as peaches and asparagus, first. Save hardier varieties, such as apples, acorn squash, or frozen goods for later in the week.

▷ Keep fruits and vegetables where you can see them. The more often you see them, the more likely you are to eat them.

▷ Keep a bowl of cut-up vegetables on the top shelf of the refrigerator.

▷ Make up a big tossed salad with several kinds of greens, cherry tomatoes, cut-up carrots, red pepper, broccoli, scallions, and sprouts. Refrigerate it in a large glass bowl with an air-tight lid, so a delicious mixed salad will be ready to enjoy for several days.

▷ Keep a fruit bowl on your kitchen counter, table, or desk at work.

▷ Pack a piece of fruit or some cut-up vegetables in your briefcase or backpack and carry moist towelettes for easy cleanup.

▷ Add fruits and vegetables to lunch by having them in soup, in salad, or cut-up raw.

▷ Increase portions when you serve vegetables. One easy way of doing this is adding fresh greens, such as Swiss chard, collards, or beet greens, to stir-fries.

▷ Add extra varieties of vegetables when you prepare soups, sauces, and casseroles. For example, add grated carrots and zucchini to spaghetti sauce.

▷ Take advantage of salad bars, which offer ready-to-eat raw vegetables and fruits, and prepared salads made with fruits and vegetables.

▷ Use vegetable-based sauces such as marinara sauce, and juices such as low-sodium V-8 or tomato juice.

▷ Choose fresh fruit for dessert. For a special dessert, try a fruit parfait with low-fat yogurt or sherbet topped with lots of berries.

▷ Freeze lots of blueberries. They make a great summer replacement for ice cream, popsicles, and other sugary foods.

▸ Key 4. Eat organic foods. In the United States, more than 1.2 billion pounds of pesticides and herbicides are sprayed on or added to food crops each year. That's roughly five pounds of pesticides for each man, woman, and child. There is a growing concern that these pesticides directly cause a significant number of cancers, and that exposure to these chemicals through food damages your body's detoxification mechanisms, thereby increasing your risk of getting cancer and other diseases. Here are my recommendations for avoiding pesticides in your diet.

▷ Do not overconsume foods that have a tendency to concentrate pesticides, such as animal fat, meat, eggs, cheese, and milk. Try to purchase free-range and organic forms of these foods.

▷ Buy organic produce, which is grown without the aid of synthetic pesticides and fertilizers. Although less than 3 percent of the total produce in the United States is grown without pesticides, organic produce is widely available.

▷ Develop a good relationship with the produce manager at your local grocery store. Explain your desire to reduce your exposure to pesticides and waxes.

▷ To remove surface pesticide residues, waxes, fungicides, and fertilizers, soak produce in a mild solution of additive-free soap, such as Ivory or pure castile soap. All-natural, biodegradable cleansers are also available at most health food stores. Spray the food with the cleanser, gently scrub, and rinse.

▶ Key 5. Reduce the intake of meat and other animal products. Study after study confirms one basic truth: the higher your intake of meat and other animal products, the higher your risk of heart disease and cancer, especially the major cancers (colon, breast, prostate, and lung cancer). There are many reasons for this association. Meat lacks the antioxidants and phytochemicals that protect us from cancer. At the same time, meat typically contains lots of saturated fat and other potentially carcinogenic compounds, including pesticide residues, heterocyclic amines, and polycyclic aromatic hydrocarbons, which form when meat is grilled, fried, or broiled. Particularly harmful to human health are cured or smoked meats, such as ham, hot dogs, bacon, and jerky, that contain sodium nitrate or sodium nitrites, which are compounds that keep food from spoiling but dramatically increase the risk of cancer. In the stomach, these chemicals react with the amino acids in foods to form highly carcinogenic compounds called nitrosamines. If you choose to eat red meat:

▷ Limit your intake to no more than 3 or 4 ounces daily—about the size of a deck of playing cards. And choose the leanest cuts available, keeping in mind that the U.S. Department of Agriculture (USDA) allows the meat and dairy industry to label fat content by weight rather than by percent of calories.

▷ Avoid consuming well-done, charbroiled, and fat-laden meats.

▷ Consider buying free-range meats or wild game.

▶ Key 6. Eat the right type of fats. It is important to consume less than 30 to 40 percent of calories as fat. However, just as important as the amount of fat is the *type* of fat you consume. The goal is to *decrease* you intake of saturated fats and of omega-6 fats found in most vegetable oils, including soy, sunflower, safflower, and corn; and *increase* the intake of monounsaturated fats from nuts, seeds, olive oil, and canola oil while ensuring an adequate intake of the omega-3 fatty acids found in fish and flaxseed oil. One diet representative of a way of eating that provides an optimal intake of the right types of fat is the traditional Mediterranean diet. See page 141 for a description.

▶ Key 7. Keep salt intake low. Too much sodium in the diet from salt (sodium chloride) can raise blood pressure in some people; it also increases that risk of cancer. In the United States, prepared foods contribute 45 percent of our sodium intake, 45 percent is added in cooking, and another 5 percent is added as a condiment. Only 5 percent of sodium intake comes from the natural ingredients in food. Here are some tips for reducing your sodium intake:

▷ Take the salt shaker off the table.

▷ Omit added salt from recipes and during food preparation.

▷ Learn to enjoy the flavors of unsalted foods.

▷ If you absolutely must have the taste of salt, try salt substitutes such as NoSalt and Nu-Salt. These products are made with potassium chloride and taste very similar to sodium chloride.

▷ Try flavoring foods with herbs, spices, and lemon juice.

▷ Choose low-salt (reduced-sodium) products when available.

▷ Read food labels carefully to determine the amounts of sodium, and learn to recognize ingredients that contain sodium. Salt, soy sauce, salt brine, or any ingredient with sodium, such as monosodium glutamate or baking soda (sodium bicarbonate), as part of its name contains sodium.

▷ In reading labels and menus, look for words that signal high sodium content, such as barbecued, broth, marinated, Parmesan, pickled, smoked, and tomato base.

▷ Prepared sauces and condiments, such as barbecue sauce, cocktail sauce, Creole sauce, mustard sauce, soy sauce, and teriyaki sauce, as well as many salad dressings, are often high in sodium.

▷ Don't eat canned foods, particularly vegetables or soups, as these are often extremely high in sodium.

STEP 7—SUPPORT YOUR BODY THROUGH PROPER NUTRITIONAL SUPPLEMENTATION AND BODY WORK

The physical care of the human body involves making sure that it has all the necessary nutritional building blocks for good health, as well as paying attention to three other important areas: exercise, breathing, and posture.

Some of these areas are described above, in other steps. I believe that there are seven keys to achieving step 7.

▶ Key 1. Take a high-potency multiple vitamin and mineral formula. To function properly, your body needs essential vitamins and minerals— each in the right amount. Vitamins and minerals function as components of enzymes, molecules that trigger and control chemical reactions. Since most enzymes in the body have both a vitamin portion and a mineral portion, it is vitally important to ensure optimal levels of these nutrients by taking a high-potency formula that provides both vitamins and minerals. (See Appendix F, "What to Look For in a Multiple Vitamin and Mineral Supplement.")

▶ Key 2. Take a pharmaceutical-grade fish oil supplement. The health benefits of the long-chain omega-3 oils from fish oils are now well known. Using a high-quality fish oil supplement is the perfect solution for people who want the health benefits of fish oils without the mercury, PCBs, dioxins, and other contaminants often found in fish. All told, about 60 different health conditions have benefited from fish oil supplementation, including diabetes, cancer, heart disease, rheumatoid arthritis and other autoimmune diseases, psoriasis, eczema, asthma, attention deficit disorder, and depression. It is estimated that fish oil supplements may reduce overall cardiovascular mortality by as much as 45 percent. For optimum benefit, take a dosage of fish oil sufficient to provide a combined total of 1,000 mg of EPA and DHA daily.

▶ Key 3. Take a "greens drink" or supplement containing concentrated sources of phytochemicals. "Greens drinks" refers to green tea and a number of commercially available products containing dehydrated barley grass, wheat grass, or algae sources such as chorella or spirulina. Such formulas are rehydrated by being mixed with water or juice. These products—which are full of phytochemicals, especially carotenes and chlorophyll—are more convenient than trying to sprout and grow your own source of greens. An added advantage is that they tend to taste better than, for example, straight wheatgrass juice.

▸ Key 4. Use appropriate natural products to deal with any "weak links." Most of us have a least one weak link that needs special attention. For one person, it might be a weak immune system. For another, it could be poor digestive function or poor circulation. Used in the context of nutritional support, many dietary supplements and herbal products have significant therapeutic effects. This book contains many examples (e.g., glucosamine sulfate for osteoarthritis, PGX for weight loss, and peppermint oil for irritable bowel syndrome) of natural products that can be at least as effective as drugs, but without the risk of serious side effects. For my other recommendations, please visit my Web site (www.doctormurray.com).

▸ Key 5. Develop and focus on your posture. Posture—how the body is held—is extremely important to good health. When the body is slouched, the shoulders are slumped, and the head is down, diaphragmatic breathing is more difficult. As a result, poor posture leads to shallow breathing and low energy. There are also possible physical results due to misalignment of vertebrae or to muscle spasms. Become aware of how you are holding your body as well as how you are breathing. When your energy is low, you will probably notice that you tend to hold your body in a tight posture with your head slightly down and your shoulders slouched. When you find yourself in this position, just start breathing with your diaphragm and pull your head up by imagining a cord affixed at the top of your head gently pulling your spine and neck straight and into alignment.

▸ Key 6. See a body worker on a regular basis. "Body work" is a general term referring to therapies involving touch, including various massage techniques, chiropractic spinal adjustment and manipulation, Rolfing, reflexology, shiatsu, and many more. All these techniques can work wonders. So, which one to choose is really a matter of personal preference. Find a technique or practitioner that you really like and incorporate body work into your routine. I have been fortunate to have experienced a broad range of body work from Rolfing and deep tissue massage to more gentle techniques like Trager massage, Feldenkais, and craniosacral therapy. My experience has led me to the conclusion that the therapist is more critical to the outcome than the technique. How do you find such a person? Word of mouth is probably the best method. Ask around.

▶ Key 7. Engage in yoga, tai chi, or stretching. These activities are very important, as they not only increase flexibility and reduce tension in the musculoskeletal system but also—once again—make us aware of our posture and breathing. As I have gotten older, I have found that stretching is even more important. As one chiropractor told me, "You are only as young as your body is flexible." If you are not familiar with stretching, you may want to take a beginners' yoga class, or pick up a video on yoga or a well-illustrated book on stretching.

FINAL COMMENTS

In the late 1970s, when I began discovering the importance of nutrition in human health, one of my heroes was Roger Williams. This brilliant man was responsible for discovering many B vitamins, including pantothenic acid and folic acid. In fact, more vitamins and their variants were discovered in his laboratory at the University of Texas than in any other laboratory in the world.

One concept that Dr. Williams introduced, which has proved to be very provocative in nutritional medicine, is "biochemical individuality." We each have unique biochemical traits that determine who we are and how we interact with the world around us. Biochemical individuality results from a combination of our genes and our environment—nature and nurture. These factors play a big role in determining how healthy we are and what ailments we are likely to experience.

Nowadays, the term "biochemical individuality" has been replaced by the term "nutrigenomics," which refers to the study of our genetic code as it relates to human nutrition. Though the term is new, the concept behind nutrigenomics clearly originated with Dr. Williams.

One major determinant of our nutrigenomic profile is a family of perhaps 100 enzymes within our cells, the cytochrome P450 enzymes. These enzymes play a critical role in detoxifying drugs, carcinogenic compounds, and hormones. Generally, each enzyme is designed to metabolize certain types of chemicals, but there is also a lot of overlap among the P450 family. This backup system ensures that your liver is usually able to detoxify your body efficiently.

Differences in the P450 enzymes can explain why some people can smoke without developing lung cancer and why some people are more susceptible than others to the harmful effects of toxic chemicals such as pesticides.

Incorporating aspects of nutrigenomics into clinical research is clarifying the effects of drugs as well as dietary practices. For example, research on the effects of coffee on heart disease has been equivocal—one study finds no correlation between coffee and hypertension; another shows a correlation with the risk of heart attack; another finds elevated cholesterol in people who drink more than four cups of coffee a day; another finds no such correlation, but only if paper filters are used. Nutrigenomics can be invaluable in clarifying these unclear relationships.

A recent study supports this notion. This study examined the association between heart attack rates and consumption of caffeine. Unlike other researchers looking into this association, these researchers also measured the activity of the liver enzyme that detoxifies caffeine—cytochrome P450 1A2 (CYP1A2). When the researchers divided the group according to whether they had a form of this enzyme that metabolizes caffeine quickly (CYP1A2*1A) or slowly (CYP1A2*1F), suddenly the picture on the impact of caffeine intake became very clear. Those whose rapid breakdown of caffeine actually decreased their risk of a heart attack by drinking coffee, but the slow caffeine metabolizers dramatically increased their risk. Drinking four cups of coffee a day was associated with a 17 percent decrease of risk in fast metabolizers and a 260 percent increase of risk in slow metabolizers.

Risk of Heart Attack and Coffee Consumption

Number of Cups Per Day	Fast Metabolizers	Slow Metabolizers
<1	1.00	1.00
1	0.48	1.24
2–3	0.57	1.67
4+	0.83	2.60

In addition to caffeine, this same enzyme system detoxifies 20 commonly prescribed drugs. There are huge variations in population groups—for example, about 50 percent of Caucasians have the slow variant compared with only 14 percent of Japanese. Researchers have found a remarkable 15-fold variation in its activity. The CYP1A2 system is also influenced by many drugs, hormones, and dietary factors. For example, it is inhibited by birth-control pills and induced by vegetables in the cabbage family. My point is that there is tremendous biochemical individuality as well as dietary and drug influences on this enzyme system—which is only one of several systems in the body that deal with detoxification reactions.

One serious drawback in conventional medical research is that it is based almost entirely on attempting to homogenize the study population. In other words, the research model assumes that we are all alike. What is becoming clearer all the time is that if researchers do not determine the genomics of their study population, the results may be compromised. Caffeine metabolism is a very good example. Meaningful results were obtained by determining the genomics of the study. If the study had been conducted in Japan without profiling caffeine metabolism, the results would probably have shown that caffeine reduced heart attack rates, since 84 percent of Japanese people rapidly metabolize caffeine. If the study had been conducted on Caucasians in the United States, it would have found no effect, because the protection experienced by fast metabolizers would have been countered by the results with the slow metabolizers.

As I hope you can now recognize, this study of coffee consumption, nutrigenomics, and heart attack rates is extremely significant and has tremendous ramifications. As my colleague Joseph Pizzorno, N.D., stated in a 2007 editorial:

> The bottom line: Current randomized clinical trial methodology is deeply flawed. Unless the study population is genetically homogeneous in the relevant biochemistry—and lifestyle factors that induce CYP activity are controlled and the participant's diet standardized—we cannot trust the results.

What Dr. Pizzorno is really saying is that although clinical trials are very important, they cannot override the individual patient's biochemistry and experience. As I have illustrated with regard to caffeine, something may help one person while harming another simply because of how each individual's own unique biochemistry responds to the substance—whether it is a drug, another chemical, or a nutrient. Through better understanding of biochemical individuality, eventually we should be able to utilize nutrition and natural medicines to an even greater extent. In the meantime, even if you are in good health, I strongly encourage you to consult a naturopathic physician. Ask for a referral or please contact:

Naturopathic Physician Associations and Referrals
American Association of Naturopathic Physicians
8201 Greensboro Drive, Suite 300
McLean, VA 22102
1-877 969-2267
Web site: www.naturopathic.org

Canadian Naturopathic Association
1255 Sheppard Ave. East
North York, Ontario M2K 1E2
Canada
(416) 496-8633
Web Site: www.naturopathicassoc.ca

If you are interested in learning more about naturopathic medicine as a career, here are the accredited schools:

Bastyr University
14500 Juanita Drive
Kenmore, WA 98028
(425) 602-3000
Web Site: www.bastyr.edu

Canadian College of Naturopathic Medicine
1255 Sheppard Avenue East
North York, Ontario M2K 1E2
Canada
(416) 498-1255
Web Site: www.ccnm.edu

National College of Naturopathic Medicine
049 S.W. Porter
Portland, OR 97201
(503) 499-4343
Web Site: www.ncnm.edu

Southwest College of Naturopathic Medicine and Health Sciences
2140 E. Broadway Road
Tempe, AZ 85282
(480) 858-9100
Web Site: www.scnm.edu

ARE YOU AN OPTIMIST?

WHAT DISTINGUISHES OPTIMISTS FROM pessimists is how they explain both good and bad events. Dr. Martin Seligman has developed a simple test to determine your level of optimism (from *Learned Optimism*, Knopf, 1981). Take as much time as you need. There are no right or wrong answers. It is important that you take the test before you read the interpretation. Read the description of each situation and vividly imagine it happening to you. Choose the response that most applies to you by circling either A or B. Ignore the letter and number codes for now; they will be explained later.

1. The project you are in charge of is a great success.   PsG

   A. *I kept a close watch over everyone's work.*   1

   B. *Everyone devoted a lot of time and energy to it.*   0

2. You and your spouse (boyfriend/girlfriend) make up after a fight.   PmG

   A. *I forgave him/her.*   0

   B. *I'm usually forgiving.*   1

3. You get lost driving to a friend's house.   PsB

   A. *I missed a turn.*   1

   B. *My friend gave me bad directions.*   0

4. Your spouse (boyfriend/girlfriend) surprises you with a gift.   PsG

   A. *He/she just got a raise at work.*   0

   B. *I took him/her out to a special dinner the night before.*   1

5. You forget your spouse's (boyfriend's/girlfriend's) birthday. PmB

    A. *I'm not good at remembering birthdays.* 1

    B. *I was preoccupied with other things.* 0

6. You get a flower from a secret admirer. PvG

    A. *I am attractive to him/her.* 0

    B. *I am a popular person.* 1

7. You run for a community office position and you win. PvG

    A. *I devote a lot of time and energy to campaigning.* 0

    B. *I work very hard at everything I do.* 1

8. You miss an important engagement. PvB

    A. *Sometimes my memory fails me.* 1

    B. *I sometimes forget to check my appointment book.* 0

9. You run for a community office position and you lose. PsB

    A. *I didn't campaign hard enough.* 1

    B. *The person who won knew more people.* 0

10. You host a successful dinner. PmG

    A. *I was particularly charming that night.* 0

    B. *I am a good host.* 1

11. You stop a crime by calling the police. PsG

    A. *A strange noise caught my attention.* 0

    B. *I was alert that day.* 1

12. You were extremely healthy all year. PsG

    A. *Few people around me were sick, so I wasn't exposed.* 0

    B. *I made sure I ate well and got enough rest.* 1

13. You owe the library $10 for an overdue book.   PmB

    A. *When I am really involved in what I am reading, I often*
    forget when it's due.   1

    B. *I was so involved in writing the report that I forgot to return*
    the book.   0

14. Your stocks make you a lot of money.   PmG

    A. *My broker decided to take on something new.*   0

    B. *My broker is a top-notch investor.*   1

15. You win an athletic contest.   PmG

    A. *I was feeling unbeatable.*   0

    B. *I train hard.*   1

16. You fail an important examination.   PsB

    A. *I wasn't as smart as the other people taking the exam.*   1

    B. *I didn't prepare for it well.*   0

17. You prepared a special meal for a friend and he / she barely
touched the food.   PvB

    A. *I wasn't a good cook.*   1

    B. *I made the meal in a rush.*   0

18. You lose a sporting event for which you have been training
for a long time.   PvB

    A. *I'm not very athletic.*   1

    B. *I'm not good at that sport.*   0

19. Your car runs out of gas on a dark street late at night.   PsB

    A. *I didn't check to see how much gas was in the tank.*   1

    B. *The gas gauge was broken.*   0

20. You lose your temper with a friend.   PmB

    A. *He/she is always nagging me.*   1

    B. *He/she was in a hostile mood.*   0

21. You are penalized for not submitting your income tax
    forms on time.   PmB

    A. *I always put off doing my taxes.*   1

    B. *I was lazy about getting my taxes done this year.* 0

22. You ask a person out on a date and he/she says no.   PvB

    A. *I was a wreck that day.*   1

    B. *I got tongue-tied when I asked him/her on the date.* 0

23. A game show host picks you out of the audience to
    participate in the show.   PsG

    A. *I was sitting in the right seat.*   0

    B. *I looked the most enthusiastic.*   1

24. You are frequently asked to dance at a party.   PmG

    A. *I am outgoing at parties.*   1

    B. *I was in perfect form that night.*   0

25. You buy your spouse (boyfriend/girlfriend) a gift he/
    she doesn't like.   PsB

    A. *I don't put enough thought into things like that.* 1

    B. *He/she has very picky tastes.*   0

26. You do exceptionally well in a job interview.   PmG

    A. *I felt extremely confident during the interview.* 0

    B. *I interview well.*   1

27. You tell a joke and everyone laughs.   PsG

   A. *The joke was funny.*   0

   B. *My timing was perfect.*   1

28. Your boss gives you too little time in which to finish a project, but you get it finished anyway.   PvG

   A. *I am good at my job.*   0

   B. *I am an efficient person.*   1

29. You've been feeling run-down lately.   PmB

   A. *I never get a chance to relax.*   1

   B. *I was exceptionally busy this week.*   0

30. You ask someone to dance and he/she says no.   PsB

   A. *I am not a good enough dancer.*   1

   B. *He/she doesn't like to dance.*   0

31. You save a person from choking to death.   PvG

   A. *I know a technique to stop someone from choking.*   0

   B. *I know what to do in crisis situations.*   1

32. Your romantic partner wants to cool things off for a while.   PvB

   A. *I'm too self-centered.*   1

   B. *I don't spend enough time with him/her.*   0

33. A friend says something that hurts your feelings.   PmB

   A. *She always blurts things out without thinking of others.*   1

   B. *My friend was in a bad mood and took it out on me.*   0

34. You employer comes to you for advice.   PvG

   A. *I am an expert in the area about which I was asked.*   0

   B. *I'm good at giving useful advice.*   1

35. A friend thanks you for helping him/her get through a bad time.   PvG

    A. *I enjoy helping him/her through tough times.*   0

    B. *I care about people.*   1

36. You have a wonderful time at a party.   PsG

    A. *Everyone was friendly.*   0

    B. *I was friendly.*   1

37. Your doctor tells you that you are in good physical shape.   PvG

    A. *I make sure I exercise frequently.*   0

    B. *I am very health-conscious.*   1

38. Your spouse (boyfriend/girlfriend) takes you away for a romantic weekend.   PmG

    A. *He/she needed to get away for a few days.*   0

    B. *He/she likes to explore new areas.*   1

39. Your doctor tells you that you eat too much sugar.   PsB

    A. *I don't pay much attention to my diet.*   1

    B. *You can't avoid sugar; it's in everything.*   0

40. You are asked to head an important project.   PmG

    A. *I just successfully completed a similar project.*   0

    B. *I am a good supervisor.*   1

41. You and your spouse (boyfriend/girlfriend) have been fighting a great deal.   PsB

    A. *I have been feeling cranky and pressured lately.*   1

    B. *He/she has been hostile lately.*   0

42. You fall down a great deal while skiing.   PmB

    A. *Skiing is difficult.*   1

    B. *The trails were icy.*   0

43. You win a prestigious award.   PvG
    A. *I solved an important problem.*   0
    B. *I was the best employee.*   1

44. Your stocks are at an all-time low.   PvB
    A. *I didn't know much about the business climate at the time.*   1
    B. *I made a poor choice of stocks.*   0

45. You win the lottery.   PsG
    A. *It was pure chance.*   0
    B. *I picked the right numbers.*   1

46. You gain weight over the holidays and you can't lose it.   PmB
    A. *Diets don't work in the long run.*   1
    B. *The diet I tried didn't work.*   0

47. You are in the hospital and few people come to visit.   PsB
    A. *I'm irritable when I am sick.*   1
    B. *My friends are negligent about things like that.*   0

48. A store won't honor your credit card.   PvB
    A. *I sometimes overestimate how much money I have.*   1
    B. *I sometimes forget to pay my credit-card bill.*   0

Scoring Key

PmB ____	PmG ____
PvB ____	PvG ____
HoB ____	
PsB ____	PsG ____
Total B ____	Total G ____
	G–B ____

INTERPRETING YOUR TEST RESULTS

The test results will give you a clue to your explanatory style. In other words, the results will tell you about how you explain things to yourself— your habit of thought. Again, remember that there are no right or wrong answers.

Your explanatory style has three crucial dimensions: permanence, pervasiveness, and personalization. Each dimension, plus a couple of others, will be scored from your test.

Permanence. When pessimists are faced with challenges or bad events, they view these events as permanent. In contrast, optimists tend to view challenges or bad events as temporary. Here are some statements that reflect the subtle differences:

Permanent (Pessimistic)	Temporary (Optimistic)
"My boss is always a jerk."	"My boss is in a bad mood today."
"You never listen."	"You are not listening."
"This bad luck will never stop."	"My luck has got to turn."

To determine how you view bad events, look at the eight items coded PmB (for "permanent bad"): 5, 13, 20, 21, 29, 33, 42, and 46. Each item with zero (0) after it is optimistic; each item followed by one (1) is pessimistic. Total the numbers at the right-hand margin of the questions coded PmB, and write the total on the PmB line on the scoring key.

If you totaled 0 or 1, you are very optimistic on this dimension; 2 or 3 is a moderately optimistic score; 4 is average; 5 or 6 is quite pessimistic; and 7 or 8 is extremely pessimistic.

Now let's take a look at the difference in explanatory style between pessimists and optimists when there is a positive event in their lives. It's just the opposite of what happened with a bad event. Pessimists view positive events as temporary; optimists view them as permanent. Here are some subtle differences in how pessimists and optimists might communicate their good fortune:

Temporary (Pessimistic)	Permanent (Optimistic)
"It's my lucky day."	"I am always lucky."
"My opponent was off today."	"I am getting better every day."
"I tried hard today."	"I always give my best."

Now total all the questions coded PmG (for "permanent good"): 2, 10, 14, 15, 24, 26, 38, and 40. Write the total on the line in the scoring key marked PmG.

If you totaled 7 or 8, you are very optimistic on this dimension; 6 is a moderately optimistic score; 4 or 5 is average; 3 is pessimistic; and 0, 1, or 2 is extremely pessimistic.

Are you starting to see a pattern? If you are scoring as a pessimist, you may want to learn how to be more optimistic. Your anxiety may be due to your belief that bad things are always going to happen, whereas good things are only a fluke.

Pervasiveness. Pervasiveness is a tendency to describe things either universal terms (everyone, always, never, etc.) rather than as specifics (a specific individual, a specific time, etc.). Pessimists tend to describe things as universals; optimists describe things as specifics.

Universal (Pessimistic)	Specific (Optimistic)
"All lawyers are jerks."	"My attorney was a jerk."
"Instruction manuals are worthless."	"This instruction manual is worthless."
"He is repulsive."	"He is repulsive to me."

Total your score for the questions coded PvB (for "pervasive bad"): 8, 17, 18, 22, 32, 44, and 48. Write the total on the PvB line.

If you totaled 0 or 1, you are very optimistic on this dimension; 2 or 3 is a moderately optimistic score; 4 is average; 5 or 6 is quite pessimistic; and 7 or 8 is extremely pessimistic.

Now let's look at the level of pervasiveness of good events. Optimists tend to view good events as universal; pessimists view them as specific. Again, this is just the opposite of how each views a bad event.

Total your score for the questions coded PvG (for "pervasive good"): 6, 7, 28, 31, 34, 35, 37, and 43. Write the total on the line labeled PvG.

If you totaled 7 or 8, you are very optimistic on this dimension; 6 is a moderately optimistic score; 4 or 5 is average; 3 is pessimistic; and 0, 1, or 2 is extremely pessimistic.

Hope. Our level of hope or hopelessness is determined by our combined level of permanence and pervasiveness. Your level of hope may be the most significant score on this test. Take your PvB and add it to your PmB score. This is your hope score.

If it is 0, 1, or 2, you are extraordinarily hopeful; 3, 4, 5, or 6 is a moderately hopeful score; 7 or 8 is average; 9, 10, or 11 is moderately hopeless; and 12, 13, 14, 15, or 16 is severely hopeless.

People who give permanent and universal explanations for their troubles tend to suffer from stress, anxiety, and depression; they tend to collapse when things go wrong. According to Dr. Seligman, no other score is as important as your hope score.

Personalization. The final aspect of explanatory style is personalization. When bad things happen, either we can blame ourselves (internalize) and lower our self-esteem as a consequence, or we can blame things beyond our control (externalize). Although it may not be right to deny personal responsibility, people who tend to externalize blame in relation to bad events have higher self-esteem and are more optimistic.

Total your score for those questions coded PsB (for "personalization bad"): 3, 9, 16, 19, 25, 30, 39, 41, and 47.

A score of 0 or 1 indicates very high self-esteem and optimism; 2 or 3 indicates moderate self-esteem; 4 is average; 5 or 6 indicates moderately low self-esteem; and 7 or 8 indicates very low self-esteem.

Now let's take a look at personalization and good events. Again, the exact opposite occurs compared with bad events. When good things happen, the person with high self-esteem internalizes whereas the person with low self-esteem externalizes.

Total your score for those questions coded PsG (for "personalization good"): 1, 4, 11, 12, 23, 27, 36, and 45. Write your score on the line marked PsG on your scoring key.

If you totaled 7 or 8, you are very optimistic on this dimension; 6 is a moderately optimistic score; 4 or 5 is average; 3 is pessimistic; and 0, 1, or 2 is extremely pessimistic.

Your Overall Scores. To compute your overall scores, first add the three B's (PmB + PvB + PsB). This is your B (bad event) score. Do the same for all the G's (PmG + PvG + PsG). This is your G score. Subtract B from G; this is your overall score.

If your B score is from 3 to 6, you are marvelously optimistic when bad events occur; 10 or 11 is average; 12 to 14 is pessimistic; anything above 14 is extremely pessimistic.

If your G score is 19 or above, you think about good events extremely optimistically; 14 to 16 is average; 11 to 13 indicates pessimism; and a score of 10 or less indicates great pessimism.

If your overall score (G minus B) is above 8, you are very optimistic across the board; if it's from 6 to 8, you are moderately optimistic; 3 to 5 is average; 1 or 2 is pessimistic; and a score of 0 or below is very pessimistic.

OSTEOPOROSIS: RISK ASSESSMENT AND RECOMMENDATIONS

CHOOSE THE ITEM IN each category that best describes you, and fill in the point value for that item in the space to the right. In categories marked with an asterisk (*), you may choose more than one item.

Frame Size	Points
Small bones or petite	10
Medium frame, very lean	5
Medium frame, average or heavy build	0
Large frame, very lean	5
Large frame, heavy build	0
Score	_____

Ethnic Background	
Caucasian	10
Asian	10
Other	0
Score	_____

Activity Level

How often do you walk briskly, jog, engage in aerobics or sports, or perform hard physical labor, for at least 30 continuous minutes?

Seldom	30
1–2 times per week	20
3–4 times per week	5
5 or more times per week	0
Score	———

Smoking

Smoke 10 or more cigarettes a day	20
Smoke fewer than 10 cigarettes a day	10
Quit smoking	5
Never smoked	0
Score	———

Personal Health Factors*

Family history of osteoporosis	20
Long-term corticosteroid use	20
Long-term anticonvulsant use	20
Drink more than 3 glasses of alcohol each week	20
Drink more than 1 cup of coffee per day	10
Seldom get outside in the sunlight	10
Score	———

For women only

Had ovaries removed	10
Premature menopause	10
Had no children	10
Score	_____

Dietary Factors

Consume more than 4 ounces of meat daily	20
Consume soft drinks regularly	20
Consume the equivalent of 3–5 servings of vegetables each day	−10
Consume at least 1 cup of green leafy vegetables each day	−10
Take 1,000 mg of supplemental calcium and 800 IU of vitamin D	−10
Consume a vegetarian diet	−10
Score	_____
Total Score	_____

INTERPRETATION

If your score is greater than 50, you are at significant risk of osteoporosis. However, you can reduce your score significantly by taking steps to reduce or eliminate risk factors. Start an exercise program; quit smoking; do not consume alcohol, coffee, or soft drinks (these leach calcium from the bones); take a good calcium and vitamin D supplement; and consume a diet low in protein and high in vegetables. These changes could take as many as 150 points off your total score.

If you are a woman, hormone replacement therapy may be appropriate for you, especially if you experienced an early menopause, had your ovaries surgically removed, or never had children. Both estrogen and progesterone have been shown to protect against bone loss. In women with established bone loss, these hormones may actually increase bone mass.

In my opinion, for women who are at risk of osteoporosis or who have already experienced significant bone loss, the benefits of natural hormone therapy (see page 107–111) outweigh the risks. But women at high risk of breast cancer or women with a disease aggravated by estrogen, such as active liver diseases or certain cardiovascular diseases, are an exception.

SUPPLEMENT RECOMMENDATIONS

- Foundation supplements

  - High-potency multiple vitamin and mineral: follow dosage recommendations on pages 299–301.

  - Greens drink: one serving daily.

  - Fish oils: 1,000 mg of EPA and DHA daily.

- Calcium: 1,200 to 1,500 mg daily.

- Vitamin D: 1,000 to 2,000 IU daily.

- Magnesium: 250 to 400 mg daily.

- Boron: 3 to 5 mg daily.

- Soy isoflavones: 90 mg daily.

APPENDIX C

HUNGER FREE
FOREVER PROGRAM

THIS IS A NEARLY effortless program for safe, effective, lifelong weight control; it was developed from major scientific discoveries regarding appetite regulation. The book *Hunger Free Forever*, which I cowrote with Michael Lyon, M.D., provides an extensive discussion of the program. My goal here is to provide some of the basic principles so you can begin to achieve your weight loss goals.

One key to the success of our program is that it promotes satiety—the state of being full or gratified to the point of satisfaction. Research has shown that humans eat to achieve satiety and those who are overweight have more frequent food cravings and a resistance to satiety after eating adequate amounts of food. Our program uncovers the reasons for cravings and resistance to satiety, and offers ways to restore normal appetite control—whether you want to lose five pounds or 200 pounds.

The Hunger Free Forever program is simple, easy to follow, and highly effective. It promotes weight loss because it is based on achieving several important goals:

- ► Decreasing appetite and calories consumed.

- ► Normalizing and stabilizing blood glucose levels.

- ► Increasing metabolism and the burning of fat, while preserving muscle mass—without the use of hazardous stimulants.

- ► Resetting the mechanisms that control the size of individual fat cells and body weight.

▶ Adjusting food and lifestyle choices to promote ideal body weight and create a healthier relationship with food.

PGX—THE SUPER-SOLUBLE FIBER

To lose weight safely, effectively, and permanently, you should greatly increase your consumption of dietary fiber. Unfortunately, to fully achieve the appetite-stabilizing effects of fiber, very large quantities of fiber must be consumed—higher quantities than most people would ever eat. Most North Americans consume 5 to 15 grams (g) of fiber per day. The USDA recommends at least 30 g per day. In reality, 75 to 100 g or more of conventional dietary fiber per day would probably be required in order to have highly significant effects on satiety in overweight individuals.

The effectiveness of fiber in reducing appetite, blood sugar, and cholesterol is directly proportional to the amount of water the fiber can absorb (its water holding capacity) and the degree of thickness or viscosity it imparts when it is in the stomach and intestine. For instance, this solubility is why oat bran lowers cholesterol and controls blood sugar better, gram for gram, than wheat bran does. With this in mind, researchers have been seeking to identify and isolate dietary fibers with the highest viscosity and water holding capacity in order to make them available as food ingredients or nutritional supplements. They have found that certain fibers, when combined, synergize and multiply one another's effects. Thus, specific fiber combinations, gram for gram, may exert health effects equivalent to larger gram quantities of similar fibers consumed alone.

Although there are many varieties of soluble fiber, a completely novel blend of soluble fibers, PolyGlycoPlex (PGX®), is the most viscous and soluble fiber ever discovered so far. The fibers in PGX work synergistically to produce a higher level of viscosity, gel-forming properties, and expansion with water than the same quantity of any other fiber alone. The blend can bind roughly hundreds of times its weight in water, resulting in a volume and viscosity three to five times greater than that of other highly soluble fibers, such as psyllium or oat beta-glucan. To put this in perspective, 5 g of PGX in a meal replacement formula or taken on its own produces a volume and viscosity that would be equal to as much as four bowls of oat bran. Thus small quantities of PGX added to foods or taken in a drink before meals will have an impact on appetite and blood sugar control equivalent to eating impractically enormous quantities of any other form of fiber.

The development of PGX is the result of intense scientific research at the University of Toronto led by Dr. David Jenkins, Dr. Tom Wolever, Dr. Alexandra Jenkins, and Dr. Vladimir Vuksan, discoverers of the now popular glycemic index (GI). My coauthor, Dr. Michael Lyon, director of the Canadian Center for Functional Medicine, then led a team of scientists for two years of exhaustive research to create the processes and formulas that led to the patent-pending ingredient PGX. Dr. Lyon continues to collaborate with the University of Toronto on PGX research. Recent studies have shown that when added to virtually any food, PGX can reduce its GI by 50 to 70 percent.

Detailed clinical studies published in major medical journals and presented at the world's major diabetes conferences have shown that PGX has the following benefits:

- Reduces appetite and promotes effective weight loss, even in the morbidly obese.

- Increases the level of compounds that block the appetite and promote satiety.

- Decreases the level of compounds that stimulate overeating.

- Reduces postprandial (after-meal) blood glucose levels when added to or taken with foods.

- Reduces the glycemic index of any food or beverage.

- Increases insulin sensitivity and decreases blood insulin levels better than any drug.

- Improves diabetes control and dramatically reduces the need for medications or insulin in diabetics.

- Stabilizes blood sugar control in the overweight and obese.

- Lowers blood cholesterol and triglycerides.

PGX—AN ABSOLUTE MUST FOR EFFECTIVE
AND PERMANENT WEIGHT LOSS

In our clinical experience, we discovered a very important fact—the key to successful weight loss is the ingestion of 2.5 to 5 g of PGX at major meals and perhaps at least twice more daily for those with an appetite more difficult to tame. Initially, we spent a lot of time in the clinic educating our patients on the importance of planning diets and menus, but then we found out that we actually got better results with our patients when we simply stressed using PGX along with becoming more conscious of what and how much they were eating.

There are various forms of PGX: capsules (either hard or soft gelatin); a zero-calorie drink mix; granules to be added to food and beverages; and a sophisticated low-carbohydrate, very low-GI meal replacement drink containing undenatured whey protein, natural flavors, and sweeteners along with vitamins and minerals. The primary supplier of PGX is Natural Factors, which offers PGX in its SlimStyles family of products for weight loss. These products can be found in health food stores throughout North America or from a number of e-tailers on the Internet. To find a store near you, please go to www.slimstyles.com. For more information about the science behind PGX go to www.PGX.com. Here is a quick checklist of how to use PGX in your daily diet:

▸ Take SlimStyles Weight Loss Drink Mix with PGX at least once per day as a meal replacement. (Note: In Canada this product is called SlimStyles Weight Loss Meal Replacement Drink Mix with PGX.)

▸ Before meals, when you are not using SlimStyles Weight Loss Drink Mix with PGX as a meal replacement, you must take PGX. If you are using PGX granules, take 2.5 to 5 g in a glass of water. (Note: SlimStyx from Natural Factors provides 2.5 g of PGX in a convenient small tube-shaped packet that is excellent to bring along with you when you are eating out. If you are using PGX in soft gelatin capsules, less PGX is required in this form. Take 2 or 3 soft gelatin capsules with a glass of water before meals.)

▸ Use PGX granules or in soft gel capsules when you are hungry between meals.

▸ Follow the menu suggestions.

▸ Drink water! It is always wise to drink at least 48 ounces of water daily, and it is vital to do so when you are taking PGX.

DIETARY SUPPLEMENTS FOR DIABETES AND HIGH BLOOD PRESSURE

SUPPLEMENT RECOMMENDATIONS FOR TYPE 2 DIABETES

The recommended supplementation program depends on the degree of blood sugar control, as indicated by self-monitored blood glucose and A_1C levels.

INITIAL SUPPLEMENTATION PROGRAMS

Level 1. Achievement of targeted blood sugar and A_1C levels <7 percent, no lipid abnormalities, no signs of complications:

- Foundation supplements

  - High-potency multiple vitamin and mineral: follow dosage recommendations on page 299–301.

  - Greens drink: one serving daily.

  - Fish oils: 1,000 mg of EPA and DHA daily.

Level 2. Failure to achieve targeted blood sugar levels, A_1C between 7 percent and 8 percent.

▸ Foundation supplements.

▸ PGX (see Appendix C): 2.5 to 5 g before or with meals.

Level 3. Failure to achieve targeted blood sugar levels, A_1C between 8 percent and 9 percent.

▸ Foundation supplements.

▸ PGX: 2.5 to 5 g before or with meals.

▸ Gymnema sylvestre extract (24 percent gymnemic acid): 200 mg twice daily.

Level 4. Failure to achieve targeted blood sugar levels, A_1C above 9 percent.

▸ Foundation supplements.

▸ PGX: 2.5 to 5 g before or with meals.

▸ Gymnema sylvestre extract (24 percent gymnemic acid): 200 mg twice daily.

▸ Mulberry extract: equivalent to 1,000 mg dried leaf three times daily.

If self-monitored blood sugar levels do not improve after four weeks of following the recommendations for the current level, move to the next highest level. For example, if you start out having an A_1C level of 8.2 percent and a fasting blood sugar level of 130 mg/dL you start on level 2 support. If after four weeks the average reading has not dropped to less than 110 mg/dL, then move to level 3 support. If blood sugar levels and A_1C levels do not reach the targeted levels with level 4 support, then a prescription medication (either an oral hypoglycemic drug or insulin) is required.

ADDITIONAL SUPPLEMENTS FOR THE PREVENTION AND TREATMENT OF DIABETIC COMPLICATIONS

With the presence of any complication add the following to the foundation supplement program (see above):

- Alpha-lipoic acid: 300 to 600 mg daily.

- Grape seed extract: 150 to 300 mg daily.

For specific complications, follow the foundation supplement program with the addition of alpha-lipoic acid and grape seed extract and add the specified supplement or supplements listed below.

For Diabetic Retinopathy

- Bilberry extract 160 to 320 mg daily. Or grape seed extract: 150 to 300 mg daily.

For Diabetic Neuropathy

- Gamma-linolenic acid from borage, evening primrose, or black currant oil: 480 mg daily.

- Capsaicin (0.075 percent) cream: apply to affected area twice daily.

For Diabetic Nephropathy

- Follow recommendations below for high blood pressure unless kidney function falls below 40 percent of normal. In that situation, do not supplement with magnesium and potassium unless advised to do so by physician.

For Poor Wound Healing

- Aloe vera gel: apply to affected areas twice daily.

For Diabetic Foot Ulcers:

▸ Ginkgo biloba extract: 120 to 240 mg daily. Or grape seed extract: 150 to 300 mg daily.

SUPPLEMENT RECOMMENDATIONS FOR HIGH BLOOD PRESSURE

For Borderline Hypertension (130–139/85–89)

Foundational supplements

Potassium chloride: 1,500 to 3,000 mg.

Magnesium: 150 to 400 mg three times daily.

PGX (see page 280 for description): 2.5 to 5 g before or with meals.

Anti-ACE fish peptides: 1,500 mg daily.

If after two months there is still no change, add celery seed extract: 150 mg daily.

For Mild (140–160/90–104) to Moderate (140–180/105–114) Hypertension

All of the above plus—

Potassium chloride: 1,500 to 3,000 mg daily.

Coenzyme Q10: 100 to 200 mg daily.

If the blood pressure has not dropped below 140/105, you will need to work with a physician to select the most appropriate medication.

For Severe Hypertension (160+/115+)

Consult a physician immediately.

All of the above for mild to moderate hypertension.

(Note: A drug may be necessary to achieve initial control. When satisfactory control over high blood pressure has been achieved, work with the physician to taper off the medication.)

GLYCEMIC INDEX, CARBOHYDRATE CONTENT, AND GLYCEMIC LOAD OF SELECTED FOODS

A COMPLETE LIST OF the glycemic index (GI) and glycemic load (GL) of all tested foods is beyond the scope of this book—it would be a book in itself. So, I have selected the most common foods. This listing will give you a general sense of what high-GL and low-GL foods are. I have listed the items by food groups, from low to high GL. You may notice that certain food groups are not listed. For example, you won't see nuts, seeds, fish, poultry, and meats listed, because these foods are so low in carbohydrates that they have little impact on blood sugar levels.

If you would like to see an even more complete listing, visit the Web site www.mendosa.com—a free site operated by the medical writer Rick Mendosa. It is an excellent resource.

FOOD	GI	CARBS, GRAMS	FIBER, GRAMS	GL
Beans (Legumes)				
Soybeans, cooked, ½ cup, 100 g	14	12	7	1.6
Peas, green, fresh, frozen, boiled, ½ cup, 80 g	48	5	2	2
White navy beans, boiled, ½ cup, 90 g	38	11	6	4.2
Kidney beans, boiled, ½ cup, 90 g	27	18	7.3	4.8
Peas, split, yellow, boiled, ½ cup, 90 g	32	16	4.7	5.1

FOOD	GI	CARBS, GRAMS	FIBER, GRAMS	GL
Lentils, ½ cup, 100g	28	19	3.7	5.3
Lima beans, baby, ½ cup cooked, 85 g	32	17	4.5	5.4
Black beans, canned, ½ cup, 95 g	45	15	7	5.7
Pinto beans, canned, ½ cup, 95 g	45	13	6.7	5.8
Chickpeas, canned, drained, ½ cup, 95 g	42	15	5	63.
Kidney beans, canned and drained, ½ cup, 95 g	52	13	7.3	6.7
Broad beans, frozen, boiled, ½ cup, 80 g	79	9	6	7.1
Peas, dried, boiled, ½ cup, 70 g	22	4	4.7	8
Baked beans, canned in tomato sauce, ½ cup, 120 g	48	21	8.8	10
Black-eyed beans, soaked, boiled, ½ cup, 120 g	42	24	5	10
Bread				
Multigrain, unsweetened, 1 slice, 30 g	43	9	1.4	4
Oat bran and honey Loaf, 1 slice, 40 g	31	14	1.5	4.5
Sourdough, rye, 1 slice, 30 g	48	12	0.4	6
Stone-ground whole wheat, 1 slice, 30 g	53	11	1.4	6
Wonder, enriched white bread, 1 slice, 20 g	73	10	0.4	7
Sourdough, wheat, 1 slice, 30 g	54	14	0.4	7.5
Pumpernickel, 1 slice, 60 g	41	21	0.5	8.6
Whole wheat, 1 slice, 35 g	69	14	1.4	9.6
Healthy Choice, hearty 7-grain, 1 slice, 38 g	56	18	1.4	10
White (wheat flour), 1 slice, 30 g	70	15	0.4	10.5
Healthy Choice, 100% whole grain, 1 slice, 38 g	62	18	1.4	11
Gluten-free multigrain, 1 slice, 35 g	79	15	1.8	12
French baguette, 30 g	95	15	0.4	14
Hamburger bun, 1 prepacked bun, 50 g	61	24	0.5	15
Rye, 1 slice, 50 g	65	23	0.4	15
Light rye, 1 slice, 50 g	68	23	0.4	16
Dark rye, black, 1 slice, 50 g	76	21	0.4	16
Croissant, 1, 50 g	67	27	0.2	18

FOOD	GI	CARBS, GRAMS	FIBER, GRAMS	GL
Kaiser roll, 1 roll, 50 g	73	25	0.4	18
Pita, 1 piece, 65 g	57	38	0.4	22
Bagel, 1, 70 g	72	35	0.4	25
Breakfast Cereals				
Oat bran, raw, 1 tablespoon, 10 g	55	7	1	4
Bran with psyllium, ⅓ cup, 30 g	47	12	12.5	5.6
Bran, ⅓ cup, 30 g	58	14	14	8
All-Bran Soy 'n' Fiber, ½ cup, 45 g	33	26	7	8.5
All-Bran, ½ cup, 40 g	42	22	6.5	9.2
Oatmeal (cooked with water), 1 cup, 245 g	42	24	1.6	10
Shredded wheat, ⅓ cup, 25 g	67	18	1.2	12
Mini Wheats (whole wheat), 1 cup, 30 g	58	21	4.4	12
All-Bran Fruit 'n' Oats, ½ cup, 45 g	39	33	6	13
Weet-Bix, 2 biscuits, 30 g	69	19	2	13
Cheerios, ½ cup, 30 g	74	20	2	15
Frosties, ¾ cup, 30 g	55	27	1	15
Corn bran, ½ cup, 30 g	75	20	1	15
Honey Smacks, ¾ cup, 30 g	56	27	1	15
Wheatbites, 30 g	72	22	2	16
Total, 30 g	76	22	2	16.7
Healthwise for Heart Health, 45 g	48	35	2	16.8
Mini Wheats (black currant) 1 cup, 30 g	71	24	2	17
Puffed wheat, 1 cup, 30 g	80	22	2	17.6
Bran Flakes, ¾ cup, 30 g	74	24	2	18
Crunchy Nut Cornflakes (Kellogg's), 30 g	72	25	2	18
Fruit Loops, 1 cup, 30 g	69	27	1	18
Cocoa Pops, ¾ cup, 30 g	77	26	1	20
Team, 30 g	82	25	1	20.5
Corn Chex, 30 g	83	25	1	20.75

FOOD	GI	CARBS, GRAMS	FIBER, GRAMS	GL
Just Right ¾ cup, 30 g	60	36	2	21.6
Corn Flakes, 1 cup, 30 g	84	26	0.3	21.8
Rice Krispies, 1 cup, 30 g	82	27	0.3	22
Rice Chex, 1 cup, 30 g	89	25	1	22
Crispix, 30 g	87	26	1	22.6
Just Right Just Grains, 1 cup, 45 g	62	38	2	23.5
Oat 'n' Honey Bake, 45 g	77	31	2	24
Raisin Bran, 1 cup, 45 g	73	35	4	25.5
Grape Nuts, ½ cup, 58 g	71	47	2	33.3
Cake				
Cake, angel food, 1 slice, 30 g	67	17	<1	11.5
Cake, sponge cake, 1 slice, 60 g	46	32	<1	14.7
Cake, cupcake, with icing and cream filling, 1	73	26	<1	19
Cake, 38 g				
Cake, chocolate fudge, mix (Betty Crocker), 73 g Cake + 33 g frosting	38	54	<1	20.5
Cake, banana cake, 1 slice, 80 g	47	46	<1	21.6
Cake, pound cake, 1 slice, 80 g	54	42	<1	22.6
Cake, French vanilla (Betty Crocker), 73 g	42	58	<1	24.4
Cake + 33 g frosting				
Cake, Lamingtons, 1, 50 g	87	29	<1	25
Cake, flan, 1 slice, 80 g	65	55	<1	35.75
Cake, scones, made from packet mix, 1 scone, 40 g	92	90	<1	83
Crackers				
Crackers, Corn Thins, puffed corn cake, 2, 12 g	87	9	<1	7.8
Crackers, Kavli, 4, 20 g	71	13	3	9.2
Crackers, Breton wheat crackers, 6, 25 g	67	14	2	9.4
Crackers, Ryvita or Wasa, 2, 20 g	69	16	3	11
Crackers, Stoned Wheat Thins, 5, 25 g	67	17	1	11.4

FOOD	GI	CARBS, GRAMS	FIBER, GRAMS	GL
Crackers, Premium soda crackers, 3, 25 g	74	17	0	12.5
Crackers, water cracker, 5, 25 g	78	18	0	14
Crackers, graham, 1, 30 g	74	22	1.4	16
Crackers, rice cake, 2, 25 g	82	21	0.4	17
Milk, Soy Milk, and Juices				
Milk, full fat, 1 cup, 250 mL	27	12	0	3
Soy, 1 cup, 250 mL	31	12	0	3.7
Milk, skim, 1 cup, 250 mL	32	13	0	4
Grapefruit juice, unsweetened, 1 cup, 250 mL	48	16	1	7.7
Nesquik chocolate powder, 3 teaspoons in 250 mL milk	55	14	0	7.7
Milk, chocolate flavored, low-fat, 1 cup, 250 mL	34	23	0	7.8
Orange juice, 1 cup, 250 mL	46	21	1	9.7
Gatorade, 1 cup, 250 mL	78	15	0	11.7
Pineapple juice, unsweetened, canned, 250 mL	46	27	1	12.4
Apple juice, unsweetened, 1 cup, 250 mL	40	33	1	13.2
Cranberry juice cocktail (Ocean Spray USA), 240 mL	68	34	0	23
Coca Cola, 375 mL	63	40	0	25.2
Soft drink, 375 mL	68	51	0	34.7
Milk, sweetened condensed, ½ cup, 160 g	61	90	0	55
Fruit				
Cherries, 20, 80 g	22	10	2.4	2.2
Plums, 3–4 small, 100 g	39	7	2.2	2.7
Peach, fresh, 1 large, 110 g	42	7	1.9	3
Apricots, fresh, 3 medium, 100 g	57	7	1.9	4
Apricots, dried, 5–6 pieces, 30 g	31	13	2.2	4
Kiwi, 1, raw, peeled, 80 g	52	8	2.4	4
Orange, 1 medium, 130 g	44	10	2.6	4.4
Peach, canned in natural juice, ½ cup, 125 g	38	12	1.5	4.5

FOOD	GI	CARBS, GRAMS	FIBER, GRAMS	GL
Pear, canned in pear juice, ½ cup, 125 g	43	13	1.5	5.5
Watermelon, 1 cup, 150 g	72	8	1	5.7
Pineapple, fresh, 2 slices, 125 g	66	10	2.8	6.6
Apple, 1 medium, 150 g	38	18	3.5	6.8
Grapes, green, 1 cup, 100 g	46	15	2.4	6.9
Apple, dried, 30g	29	24	3.0	6.9
Prunes, pitted (Sunsweet), 6, 40 g	29	25	3.0	7.25
Pear, fresh, 1 medium, 150 g	38	21	3.1	8
Fruit cocktail, canned in natural juice, ½ cup, 125 g	55	15	1.5	8.25
Apricots, canned, light syrup, ½ cup, 125 g	64	13	1.5	8.3
Peach, canned, light syrup, ½ cup, 125 g	52	18	1.5	9.4
Mango, 1 small, 150 g	55	19	2.0	10.4
Figs, dried, tenderized (water added), 50 g	61	22	3.0	13.4
Sultanas, ¼ cup, 40 g	56	30	3.1	16.8
Banana, raw, 1 medium, 150 g	55	32	2.4	17.6
Raisins, ¼ cup, 40 g	64	28	3.1	18
Dates, dried, 5, 40 g	103	27	3.0	27.8
Grains				
Rice bran, extruded, 1 tablespoon, 10 g	19	3	1	0.57
Barley, pearled, boiled, ½ cup, 80 g	25	17	6	4.25
Millet, cooked, ½ cup, 120 g	71	12	1	8.52
Bulgur, cooked, ⅔ cup, 120 g	48	22	3.5	10.6
Brown rice, steamed, 1 cup, 150 g	50	32	1	16
Couscous, cooked, ⅔ cup, 120 g	65	28	1	18
Rice, white, boiled, 1 cup, 150 g	72	36	0.2	26
Rice, arborio risotto rice, white, boiled, 1 cup, 100 g	69	35	0.2	29
Rice, basmati, white, boiled, 1 cup, 180 g	58	50	0.2	29

FOOD	GI	CARBS, GRAMS	FIBER, GRAMS	GL
Buckwheat, cooked, ½ cup, 80 g	54	57	3.5	30
Rice, instant, cooked, 1 cup, 180 g	87	38	0.2	33
Tapioca (steamed 1 hour), 100 g	70	54	<1	38
Tapioca (boiled with milk), 1 cup, 265 g	81	51	<1	41
Rice, jasmine, white, long-grain, steamed, 1 cup, 180 g	109	39	0.2	42.5
Ice Cream				
Ice cream, low-fat French vanilla, 100 mL	38	15	0	5.7
Ice cream, full fat, 2 scoops, 50 g	61	10	0	6.1
Jam				
Jam, no sugar, 1 tablespoon, 25 g	55	11	<1	6
Jam, sweetened, 1 tablespoon	48	17	<1	8
Muffins and Pancakes				
Muffins, chocolate butterscotch, from mix, 1, 50 g	53	28	1	15
Muffins, apple, oat, and sultana, from mix, 1, 50 g	54	28	1	15
Muffins, apricot, coconut, and honey, from mix, 1, 50 g	60	27	1.5	16
Muffins, banana, oat, and honey, from mix, 1, 50 g	65	28	1.5	18
Muffins, apple, 1, 80 g	44	44	1,5	19
Muffins, bran, 1, 80 g	60	34	2.5	20
Muffins, blueberry, 1, 80 g	59	41	1,5	24
Pancake, buckwheat, from dry mix, 1, 40 g	102	30	2	30
Pancakes, from dry mix, 1 large, 80 g	67	58	1	39
Pasta				
Pasta, tortellini, cheese, cooked, 180 g	50	21	2	10.5
Pasta, ravioli, meat-filled, cooked, 1 cup, 220 g	39	30	2	11.7
Pasta, vermicelli, cooked, 1 cup, 180 g	35	45	2	15.7

FOOD	GI	CARBS, GRAMS	FIBER, GRAMS	GL
Pasta, rice noodles, fresh, boiled, 1 cup, 176 g	40	44	0.4	17.6
Pasta, spaghetti, whole-meal, cooked, 1 cup, 180 g	37	48	3.5	17.75
Pasta, fettuccine, cooked, 1 cup, 180 g	32	57	2	18.2
Pasta, spaghetti, gluten-free in tomato sauce, 1 small tin, 220 g	68	27	2	18.5
Pasta, macaroni and cheese, packaged, cooked, 220 g	64	30	2	19.2
Pasta, star pastina, cooked, 1 cup, 180 g	38	56	2	21
Pasta, spaghetti, white, cooked, 1 cup, 180 g	41	56	2	23
Pasta, rice pasta, brown, cooked, 1 cup, 180 g	92	57	2	52
Sugars				
Fructose, 10 g	23	10	0	2.3
Honey, ½ tablespoon, 10 g	58	16	0	4.6
Lactose, 10 g	46	10	0	4.6
Sucrose, 10 g	65	10	0	6.5
Glucose, 10 g	102	10	0	10.2
Maltose, 10 g	105	10	0	10.5
Snacks				
Corn chips, Doritos original, 50 g	42	33	<1	13.9
Snickers, 59 g	41	35	0	14.3
Tofu frozen dessert (nondairy), 1, 100 g	115	13	<1	15
Real Fruit bars, strawberry, 20 g	90	17	<1	15.3
Twix cookie bar (caramel), 59 g	44	37	<1	16.2
Pretzels, 50 g	83	22	<1	18.3
Mars bar, 60 g	65	41	0	26.6
Skittles, 62 g	70	55	0	38.5
Soups				
Tomato, canned, 220 mL	38	15	1.5	6

FOOD	GI	CARBS, GRAMS	FIBER, GRAMS	GL
Black bean, 220 mL	64	9	3.4	6
Lentil, canned, 220 mL	44	14	3	6
Split pea, canned, 220 mL	60	13	3	8
Vegetables				
Carrots, raw, 1/2 cup, 80 g	16	6	1.5	1
Low glycemic vegetables:	≈20	≈7	≈1.5	≈1.4
Asparagus, 1 cup cooked or raw				
Bell peppers, 1 cup cooked or raw				
Broccoli, 1 cup cooked or raw				
Brussels sprouts, 1 cup cooked or raw				
Cabbage, 1 cup cooked or raw				
Cauliflower, 1 cup cooked or raw				
Cucumber, 1 cup				
Celery, 1 cup cooked or raw				
Eggplant, 1 cup				
Green beans, 1 cup cooked or raw				
Kale, 1 cup cooked, 2 cups raw				
Lettuce, 2 cups raw				
Mushrooms, 1 cup				
Spinach, 1 cup cooked, 2 cups raw				
Tomatoes, 1 cup				
Zucchini, 1 cup cooked or raw				
Carrots, peeled, boiled, ½ cup, 70 g	49	3	1.5	1.5
Beets, canned, drained, 2–3 slices, 60 g	64	5	1	3
Pumpkin, peeled, boiled, ½ cup, 85 g	75	6	3.4	4.5
Parsnips, boiled, ½ cup, 75 g	97	8	3	8
Sweet corn on the cob, boiled 20 minutes, 80 g	48	14	2.9	8
Corn, canned and drained, ½ cup, 80 g	55	15	3	8.5
Sweet potato, peeled, boiled, 80 g	54	16	3.4	8.6

FOOD	GI	CARBS, GRAMS	FIBER, GRAMS	GL
Sweet corn, ½ cup boiled, 80 g	55	18	3	10
Potatoes, peeled, boiled, 1 medium, 120 g	87	13	1.4	10
Potatoes, with skin, boiled, 1 medium, 120 g	79	15	2.4	11
Yam, boiled, 80 g	51	26	3.4	13
Potatoes, baked in oven (no fat), 1 medium, 120 g	93	15	2.4	14
Potatoes, mashed, ½ cup, 120 g	91	16	1	14
Potatoes, instant potato, prepared, ½ cup	83	18	1	15
Potatoes, new, unpeeled, boiled, 5 small (cocktail), 175 g	78	25	2	20
Cornmeal (polenta), ⅓ cup, 40 g	68	30	2	20
Potatoes, french fries, fine-cut, small serving, 120g	75	49	1	36
Gnocchi, cooked, 1 cup, 145 g	68	71	1	48
Yogurt				
Yogurt, low-fat, artificial sweetener, 200 g	14	12	0	2
Yogurt, with fruit, 200 g	26	30	0	8
Yogurt, low-fat, 200 g	33	26	0	8.5

WHAT TO LOOK FOR IN A MULTIPLE VITAMIN AND MINERAL SUPPLEMENT

A HEALTH-PROMOTING DIET IS an essential component of good health, and so too is proper nutritional supplementation. Some experts say that theoretically you can meet all your nutritional needs through diet alone, but in reality most Americans do not come anywhere near the optimal levels. In an effort to increase their intake of essential nutrients, many Americans look to vitamin and mineral supplements.

Current estimates are that more than 70 percent of Americans now regularly take vitamin or mineral supplements. It seems that taking vitamin and mineral supplements has become a way of life for most Americans. Sixty-seven percent of people who use supplements take only one; the majority of these (46 percent) take a multiple vitamin and mineral product. Unfortunately, most people who take a multiple vitamin and mineral formulas are still not getting what they really need, because they are being misled: they think that the "one a day" multiple vitamin is meeting all their needs for optimum nutrition.

GIVING YOUR BODY THE TOOLS IT NEEDS

For optimum health, a high-quality multiple vitamin and mineral supplement is an absolute necessity. A high-quality multiple is one that provides optimal levels of both vitamins and minerals. Your body needs all the important building blocks in order to achieve health. The following recommendations provide an optimum intake range to guide you in selecting a high-quality multiple. (Note that different vitamins and minerals are measured in different units. IU = international units; mg = milligrams μg = micrograms.)

Vitamin	Range for Adults
Vitamin A (retinol)*	2,500–5,000 IU
Vitamin A (from beta-carotene)	5000–25,000 IU
Vitamin B$_1$ (thiamin)	10–100 mg
Vitamin B$_2$ (riboflavin)	10–50 mg
Vitamin B$_3$ (niacin)	10–100 mg
Vitamin B$_5$ (pantothenic acid)	25–100 mg
Vitamin B$_6$ (pyridoxine)	25–100 mg
Vitamin B$_{12}$ (cobalamin)	400 μg
Vitamin C (ascorbic acid)	250–500 mg
Vitamin D†	100–600 IU
Vitamin E (d-alpha tocopherol)	100–400 IU
Niacinamide	10–30 mg
Biotin	100–600 μg
Folic acid	400–800 μg
Choline	10–100 mg
Inositol	10–100 mg

* Women of childbearing age who may become pregnant should not take more than 2,500 IU of retinol daily, owing to the possible risk of birth defects. (Note: Beta-carotene is safe during pregnancy and lactation.)
† People living in northern latitudes should supplement at the high range.

Mineral	Range for Adults
Calcium*	250–1,000 mg
Chromium	200–400 µg
Copper	1–2 mg
Iodine	50–150 µg
Iron†	15–30 mg
Magnesium	250–350 mg
Manganese	3–5 mg
Molybdenum	10–25 µg
Selenium	100–200 µg
Silica	1–25 mg
Vanadium	50–100 µg
Zinc	15–20 mg

*Women should take 800 to 1,000 mg of calcium to reduce the risk of osteoporosis.
† Men and postmenopausal women rarely need supplemental iron.

To find a multiple vitamin and mineral formula that meet these criteria, read labels carefully. Be aware that you will not be able to find a formula that can provide all of these nutrients at these levels in one single pill—such a pill would simply be too large. Usually, at least four to six tablets will be required to meet these levels. Although many "one-a-day" supplements provide good levels of vitamins, they are woefully insufficient in the levels of minerals.

REALISTIC EXPECTATIONS

In addition to the large number of studies showing benefits from the individual nutrients in a high-potency multiple, studies have shown that people taking a multiple vitamin and mineral formula may have higher energy, improved brain function, fewer colds or infections, an improved ability to deal with stress, a greater sense of well-being, and other health benefits. Still, many people taking a multiple may feel nothing. But not feeling anything doesn't mean that the higher nutrient levels you are ingesting are not being used by your body. For example, there is evidence that people taking nutritional supplements may have a lowered risk of heart disease, cancer, cataracts, and some degenerative diseases. In one large study it was found that women taking a multiple vitamin and mineral formula for more than 14 years had a 75 percent reduced rate of colon cancer. It is extremely unlikely that these women felt the impressive protection they were being given by their supplement; nonetheless, they definitely realized the benefits.

NOTES

THE PRIMARY RESOURCES FOR the materials presented in this book are from my personal files. Over the past 30 years, I have painstakingly collected from medical journals thousands of scientific articles on the healing power of foods and food components. The references provided are by no means intended to represent a complete reference list for all the studies reviewed or mentioned in this book. Instead, I have chosen to focus on key studies and comprehensive review articles that readers, especially medical professionals, may find helpful.

I encourage interested readers to visit the Web site of the National Library of Medicine (NLM) at http://gateway.nlm.nih.gov for additional studies. The NLM Gateway is a web-based system that lets users search simultaneously in multiple retrieval systems. From this site you can access all the NLM databases, including PubMed. The PubMed database was developed in conjunction with publishers of biomedical literature as a search tool for accessing literature citations and linking to full-text journal articles at Web sites of participating publishers. Publishers participating in PubMed supply NLM with their citations electronically prior to or at the time of publication. If the publisher has a Web site that offers full texts of its journals, PubMed provides links to that site, as well as to sites with other biological data, sequence centers, etc. User registration, a subscription fee, or some other type of fee may be required to access the full text of articles in some journals.

PubMed provides access to bibliographic information, including MEDLINE—the NLM's premier bibliographic database covering the fields of medicine, nursing, dentistry, veterinary medicine, the health care system, and the preclinical sciences. MEDLINE contains bibliographic citations and author abstracts from more than 4,000 medical journals published in the

United States and 70 other countries. The file contains more than 11 million citations dating back to the mid-1960s. Coverage is worldwide, but most records are from English-language sources or have English abstracts (summaries). Conducting a search is quite easy, and the site has a link to a tutorial that fully explains the search process.

1. A Matter of Trust—Making Medicine or Making Money?

1. M. A. Gagnon and J. Lexchin, "The Cost of Pushing Pills: A New Estimate of Pharmaceutical Promotion Expenditures in the United States," *Public Library Science Med* 5(1) (2008): e1.

2. General Accountability Office, "Prescription Drugs: FDA Oversight of Direct-to-Consumer Advertising has limitations" (2002), http://www.gao.gov/new.items/d03177.pdf.

3. M. Angell, *The Truth about the Drug Companies: How They Deceive Us and What to Do about It* (New York: Random House, 2004).

4. J. Alvorn, *Powerful Medicines: The Benefits, Risks, and Costs of Prescription Drugs* (New York: Vintage, 2005.)

5. S. E. Nissen and K. Wolski, "Effect of Rosiglitazone on the Risk of Myocardial Infarction and Death from Cardiovascular Causes," *N Engl J Med* 356(26) (2007): 2457–2471.

6. L. L. Leape, "Unnecessary Surgery," *Health Serv Res* 24 (1989): 351–407.

7. T. B. Graboys, B. Biegelsen, S. Lampert, et al., "Results of a Second-Opinion Trial among Patients Recommended for Coronary Angiography," *JAMA* 268(18) (1992): 2537–2540.

8. R. Moynihan and A. Cassells, *Selling Sickness: How the World's Biggest Pharmaceutical Companies Are Turning Us All into Patients* (New York: Nations, 2005).

9. See http://www.nhlbi.nih.gov/guidelines/cholesterol/atp3upd04_disclose.htm accessed 2/08/08.

10. R. Smith, "Medical Journals Are an Extension of the Marketing Arm of Pharmaceutical Companies," *Public Library Science Med* 2 (2005): 364–366.

11. R. Horton, "The Dawn of McScience," *New York Rev Books* 51 (2004): 7–9.

12. "Peer Review Congress," *JAMA* 287(21) (2002): 2749–2898.

13. P. C. Gøtzsche, A. Hróbjartsson, H. K. Johansen, et al., "Ghost Authorship in Industry-Initiated Randomised trials," *Public Library Science Med* 4(1) (2007): e19.

14. T. Bodenheimer, "Uneasy Alliance—Clinical Investigators and the Pharmaceutical Industry," *N Engl J Med* 342(20) (2000): 1539–1544.

15. M. Shuchman, "Commercializing Clinical Trials—Risks and Benefits of the CRO Boom," *N Engl J Med* 357(14) (2007): 1365–1368.

16. J. Berg Hrachovec and M. Mora, "Reporting of 6-Month versus 12-Month Data in a Clinical Trial of Celecoxib," *JAMA* 286(19) (2001): 2398.

17. J. M. Wright, T. L. Perry, K. L. Bassett, and G. K. Chambers, "Reporting of 6-Month versus 12-Month Data in a Clinical Trial of Celecoxib," *JAMA* 286(19) (2001): 2398–2400.

18. M. A. Steinman, L. A. Bero, M. M. Chren, and C. S. Landefeld, "Narrative Review: The Promotion of Gabapentin—An Analysis of Internal Industry Documents," *Ann Intern Med* 145 (2006): 284–293.

19. G. P. Oakley, "Folic Acid—Preventable Spina Bifida and Anencephaly," *JAMA* 269 (1993): 1292–1293.

20. T. J. Moore, B. M. Psaty, and C. D. Furberg, "Time to Act on Drug Safety," *JAMA* 279(19) (1998): 1571–1573.

21. M. M. Wolfe, D. R. Lichtenstein, and G. Singh, "Gastrointestinal Toxicity of Nonsteroidal Anti-Inflammatory Drugs," *N Engl J Med* 340 (1999): 1888–1889.

L. M. Verbrugge and D. L. Patrick, "Seven Chronic Conditions: Their Impact on U.S. Adults' Activity Levels and Use of Medical Services," *Am J Public Health* 85(2) (1995): 173–182.

W. T. M. Oojendijk, J. P. Mackenbach, and H. H. B. Limberger, *What Is Better? An Investigation into the Use [of] and Satisfaction with Complementary and Official Medicine in the Netherlands* (Rotterdam Institute of Preventive Medicine and the Technical Industrial Organization, 1980).

2. The Number One Thing That They Don't Want You to Know

1. B. Klopfer, "Psychological Variables in Human Cancer," *J Proj Tech* 21 (1957): 331–340.

2. F. Benedetti, "Mechanisms of Placebo and Placebo-Related Effects across Diseases and Treatments," *Annu Rev Pharmacol Toxicol* 48 (2008): 33–60.

3. D. D. Price, D. G. Finniss, and F. Benedetti, "A Comprehensive Review of the Placebo Effect: Recent Advances and Current Thought," *Annu Rev Psychol* 59 (2008): 565–590.

4. H. K. Beecher, "The Powerful Placebo," *JAMA* 159 (1955): 1602–1606.

5. H. Benson and R. Friedman, "Harnessing the Power of the Placebo Effect and Renaming It 'Remembered Wellness,' " *Annu Rev Med* 47 (1996): 193–199.

6. F. Benedetti, M. Lanotte, L. Lopiano, and L. Colloca, "When Words Are Painful: Unraveling the Mechanisms of the Nocebo Effect," *Neuroscience* 147(2) (2007): 260–271.

7. B. Olshansky, "Placebo and Nocebo in Cardiovascular Health: Implications for Healthcare, Research, and the Doctor-Patient Relationship," *J Am Coll Cardiol* 49(4) (2007): 415–421.

8. D. P. O'Hara, "Is There a Role for Prayer and Spirituality in Health Care? *Med Clin North Am* 86(1) (2002): 33–46.

9. L. Pizzorno, "Spirituality and Healing," *A Textbook of Natural Medicine*, ed. J. E. Pizzorno and M. T. Murray, 519–532 (London: Churchill-Livingston, 2005).

10. T. McNichol, "The New Faith in Medicine," *USA Today* (April 7, 1996): 4.

11. H. Benson, "The Relaxation Response: Therapeutic Effect," *Science* 278 (1997): 1694–1751.

12. J. Levin, "Spiritual Determinants of Health and Healing: An Epidemiologic Perspective on Salutogenic Mechanisms," *Altern Ther Health Med* 9(6) (2003): 48–57.

3. An Overlooked Goal of Healing—Removing Obstacles to a Cure

1. J. A. LeClair and D. W. Quig, "Mineral Status, Toxic Metal Exposure, and Children's Behaviour," *Orthomolecular Med* 16 (2001): 13–32.

2. R. Tuthill, "Hair Lead Levels Related to Children's Classroom Attention-Deficit Behavior," *Arch Environ Health* 51 (1996): 214–220.

3. C. Moon and M. Marlow, "Hair-Aluminum Concentrations and Children's Classroom Behavior," *Biol Trace Elem Res* 11 (1986): 5–12.

4. Y. Cheng, J. Schwartz, D. Sparrow, et al., "Bone Lead and Blood Lead Levels in Relation to Baseline Blood Pressure and the Prospective Development of Hypertension: The Normative Aging Study," *Am J Epidemiol* 153(2) (2001): 164–171.

5. I. Hertz-Picciotto and J. Croft, "Review of the Relation between Blood Lead and Blood Pressure," *Epidemiol Rev* 15(2) 1993: 352–373.

6. G. Vivoli, M. Bergomi, P. Borella, et al., "Cadmium in Blood Urine, and Hair Related to Human Hypertension," *J Trace Elem Electrolytes Health Dis* 3(3) (1989): 139–145.

7. D. A. Bass, D. Hickock, D. Quig, and K. Urek, "Trace Element Analysis in Hair: Factors Determining Accuracy, Precision, and Reliability," *Altern Med Rev* 6(5) (2001): 472–481.

8. B. C. Sirois and M. M. Burg, "Negative Emotion and Coronary Heart Disease: A Review," *Behav Modif* 27(1) (2003) 83–102.

9. L. D. Kubzansky and I. Kawachi, "Going to the Heart of the Matter: Do Negative Emotions Cause Coronary Heart Disease?" *J Psychosom Res* 48(4–5) (2000): 323–337.

10. M. M. Müller, H. Rau, S. Brody, et al., "The Relationship between Habitual Anger Coping Style and Serum Lipid and Lipoprotein Concentrations," *Biol Psychol* 41(1) (1995): 69–81.

11. L. D. Kubzansky, "Sick at Heart: The Pathophysiology of Negative Emotions," *Cleve Clin J Med* 74(Suppl. 1) (2007): S69–S72.

12. J. K. Kiecolt-Glaser, L. McGuire, T. F. Robles, and R. Glaser, "Emotions, Morbidity, and Mortality: New Perspectives from Psychoneuroimmunology," *Annu Rev Psychol.* 53 (2002): 83–107.

4. Functional Medicine versus the Treatment of Disease

1. J. E. Richter, P. J. Kahrilas, J. Johanson, et al., "Efficacy and Safety of Esomeprazole Compared with Omeprazole in GERD Patients with Erosive Esophagitis: A Randomized Controlled Trial," *Am J Gastroenterol* 96(3) (2001): 656–665.

2. P. J. Kahrilas, G. W. Falk, D. A. Johnson, et al., "Esomeprazole Improves Healing and Symptom Resolution as Compared with Omeprazole in Reflux Oesophagitis Patients: A Randomized Controlled Trial, the Esomeprazole Study Investigators," *Aliment Pharmacol Ther* 14(10) (2000): 1249–1258.

3. T. Lind, L. Rydberg, A. Kylebäck, et al., "Esomeprazole Provides Improved Acid Control versus Omeprazole in Patients with Symptoms of Gastro-Oesophageal Reflux Disease," *Aliment Pharmacol Ther* 14(7) (2000): 861–867.

4. A. Berenson, "Where Has All the Prilosec Gone?" *New York Times* (March 2, 2005), http://www.nytimes.com/2005/03/02/business/02prilosec.html? pagewanted=print&position=.

5. U. Stiefel, R. L. Jump, and C. J. Donskey, "Suppression of Gastric Acid Production by Proton Pump Inhibitor Treatment Facilitates Colonization of the Large Intestine by Vancomycin-Resistant *Enterococcus* and *Klebsiella pneumoniae* in Clindamycin-Treated Mice," *Antimicrob Agents Chemother* 50(11) (2006): 3905–3907.

6. S. Dial, J. A. Delaney, A. N. Barkun, and S. Suissa, "Use of Gastric Acid-Suppressive Agents and the Risk of Community-Acquired *Clostridium difficile*-Associated Disease," *JAMA* 294(23) (December 21, 2005): 2989–2995.

7. J. A. Hawrelak, "Probiotics," in *A Textbook of Natural Medicine*, ed. J. E. Pizzorno and M. T. Murray (London: Churchill-Livingston, 2005), 1995–1216.

8. F. Yan and D. B. Polk, "Probiotics as Functional Food in the Treatment of Diarrhea," *Curr Opin Clin Nutr Metab Care* 9(6) (2006): 717–721.

9. A. Sullivan and C. E. Nord, "Probiotics and Gastrointestinal Diseases," *J Intern Med* 257(1) (2005): 78–92.

10. D. Lesbros-Pantoflickova, I. Corthésy-Theulaz, and A. L. Blum, "*Helicobacter pylori* and Probiotics," *J Nutr* 137 (Suppl. 2) (2007): 812S–818S.

11. J. R. Lambert and P. Midolo, "The Actions of Bismuth in the Treatment of *Helicobacter pylori* Infection," *Aliment Pharmacol Ther* 11(Suppl. 1) (1997): 27–33.

12. R. J. Laheij, M. C. Sturkenboom, R. J. Hassing, et al., "Risk of Community-Acquired Pneumonia and Use of Gastric Acid-Suppressive Drugs," *JAMA* 292 (October 27, 2004): 1955–1960.

13. R. J. Valuck and J. M. Ruscin, "A Case-Control Study on Adverse Effects: H2 Blocker or Proton Pump Inhibitor Use and Risk of Vitamin B$_{12}$ Deficiency in Older Adults," *J Clin Epidemiol* 57 (4) (April 2004): 422–428.

14. M. Wolters, A. Strohle, and A. Hahn, "Cobalamin: A Critical Vitamin in the Elderly," *Prev Med* 29(6) (2004): 1256–1266.

15. T. Fukai, A. Marumo, K. Kaitou, et al., "Anti-*Helicobacter pylori* Flavonoids from Licorice Extract," *Life Sci* 71 (2002): 1449–1463.

16. V. Balakrishnan, M. V. Pillai, P. M. Raveendran, et al., "Deglycyrrhizinated Liquorice in the Treatment of Chronic Duodenal Ulcer," *J Assoc Physicians India*. 26 (1978): 811–814.

17. A. G. Morgan, W. A. McAdam, C. Pacsoo, et al. "Comparison between Cimitidine and Caved-S in the Treatment of Gastric Ulceration, and Subsequent Maintenance Therapy," *Gut* 23 (1982): 545–551.

18. B. Kligler and S. Chaudhary, "Peppermint Oil," *Am Fam Physician* 75(7) (2007): 1027–1030.

19. B. May, S. Kohler, and B. Schneider, "Efficacy and Tolerability of a Fixed Combination of Peppermint Oil and Caraway Oil in Patients Suffering from Functional Dyspepsia," *Aliment Pharmacol Ther* 14 (2000): 1671–1677.

20. G. Iacono, F. Cavataio, G. Montalto, et al., "Intolerance of Cow's Milk and Chronic Constipation in Children," *N Engl J Med* 339(16) (1998) 1100–1104.

5. Is Symptom Relief a Path to Bad Medicine?

1. N. T. Mathew, "Chronic Refractory Headache," *Neurology* 43 (Suppl. 3) (1993): S26–S33.

2. E. L. Hurwitz, P. D. Aker, A. H. Adams, et al., "Manipulation and Mobilization of the Cervical Spine: A Systematic Review of Literature," *Spine* 21 (1996): 1746–1760.

3. M. Haas, G. Bronfort, and R. L. Evans, "Chiropractic Clinical Research: Progress and Recommendations," *J Manipulative Physiol Ther* 29(9) (2006): 695–706.

4. D. M. Biondi, "Physical Treatments for Headache: A Structured Review," *Headache* 45(6) (2005): 738–746.

5. M. L. Lenssinck, L. Damen, A. P. Verhagen, et al., "The Effectiveness of Physiotherapy and Manipulation in Patients with Tension-Type Headache: A Systematic Review," *Pain* 112(3) (2004): 381–388.

6. B. Larsson and J. Carlsson, "A School-Based, Nurse-Administered Relaxation Training for Children with Chronic Tension-Type Headache," *J Pediatr Psychol* 21 (1996): 603–614.

7. B. Larsson, J. Carlsson, A. Fichtel, and L. Melin, "Relaxation Treatment of Adolescent Headache Sufferers: Results from a School-Based Replication Series," *Headache.* 45(6) (2005): 692–704.

8. K. A. Holroyd and J. B. Drew, "Behavioral Approaches to the Treatment of Migraine," *Semin Neurol* 26(2) (2006): 199–207.

9. J. C. Rains, D. B. Penzien, D. C. McCrory, and R. N. Gray, "Behavioral Headache Treatment: History, Review of the Empirical Literature, and Methodological Critique," Headache 45(Suppl. 2) (2005): S92–S109.

10. L. E. Mansfield, T. R. Vaughan, S. F. Waller, et al., "Food Allergy and Adult Migraine: Double-Blind and Mediator Confirmation of an Allergic Etiology," *Ann Allergy* 55 (1985): 126–129.

11. C. M. Carter, J. Egger, and J. F. Soothill, "A Dietary Management of Severe Childhood Migraine," *Hum Nutr Appl Nutr* 39 (1985): 294–303.

12. E. C. Hughes, P. S. Gott, R. C. Weinstein, and R. Binggeli, "Migraine: A diagnostic Test for Etiology of Food Sensitivity by a Nutritionally Supported Fast and Confirmed by Long-Term Report," *Ann Allergy* 55 (1985): 28–32.

13. J. Egger, C. M. Carter, J. Wilson, et al., "Is Migraine Food Allergy? A Double-Blind Controlled Trial of Oligoantigenic Diet Treatment," *Lancet* 2 (1983): 865–869.

14. J. Monro, J. Brostoff, C. Carini, and K. Zilkha, "Food Allergy in Migraine: Study of Dietary Exclusion and RAST," *Lancet* 2 (1980): 1–4.

15. J. Schoenen, J. Jacquy, and M. Lenaerts, "Effectiveness of High-Dose Riboflavin in Migraine Prophylaxis: A Randomized Controlled Trial," *Neurology* 50 (1998): 466–470.

16. D. R. Swanson, "Migraine and Magnesium: Eleven Neglected Connections," *Perspect Biol Med* 31 (1998): 526–557.

17. A. Mauskop and B. M. Altura, "Role of Magnesium in the Pathogenesis and Treatment of Migraines," *Clin Neurosci* 5 (1998): 24–27.

18. V. Pfaffenrath, P. Wessely, C. Meyer, et al., "Magnesium in the Prophylaxis of Migraine—A double-Blind Placebo-Controlled Study," *Cephalalgia* 16 (1996): 436–440.

19. A. Peikert, C. Wilimzig, and R. Kohne-Volland, "Prophylaxis of Migraine with Oral Magnesium: Results from a Prospective, Multi-Center, Placebo-Controlled and Double-Blind Randomized Study," *Cephalalgia* 16 (1996): 257–263.

20. R. Agosti, R. K. Duke, J. E. Chrubasik, and S. Chrubasik, "Effectiveness of *Petasites hybridus* Preparations in the Prophylaxis of Migraine: A Systematic Review," *Phytomedicine* 13(9–10) (2006): 743–746.

21. M. Grossman and H. Schmidramsl, "An Extract of *Petasites hybridus* Is Effective in the Prophylaxis of Migraine," *Int J Clin Pharm* 38 (2000): 430–435.

22. F. Marra, L. Lynb, M. Coombes, et al., "Does Antibiotic Exposure during Infancy Lead to Development of Asthma? A Systematic Review and Meta-Analysis," *Chest* 129 (2006): 610–618.

23. S. S. Braman, "Chronic Cough Due to Acute Bronchitis: ACCP Evidence-Based Clinical Practice Guidelines," *Chest* 129(Suppl. 1) (2006): 95S–103S.

24. R. Gonzales and M. Sande, "What Will It Take to Stop Physicians from Prescribing Antibiotics in Acute Bronchitis?" *Lancet* 345(8951) (1995): 665–666.

25. J. Froom, L. Culpepper, M. Jacobs, et al., "Antimicrobials for Acute Otitis Media? A Review from the International Primary Care Network," *Br Med J* 315 (1997): 98–102.

26. C. Del Mar, P. Glasziou, and M. Hayem, "Are Antibiotics Indicated as Initial Treatment for Children with Acute Otitis Media? A Meta-Analysis," *BMJ* 314 (7093) (1997): 1526–1529.

27. P. P. Glasziou, C. B. Del Mar, S. L. Sanders, and M. Hayem, "Antibiotics for Acute Otitis Media in Children," *Cochrane Database Syst Rev* 1 (2004): CD000219.

28. P. B. Van Cauwenberge, "The Role of Allergy in Otitis Media with Effusion," *Ther Umschau* 39 (1982): 1011–1016.

29. P. Bellionin, A. Cantani, and F. Salvinelli, "Allergy: A Leading Role in Otitis Media with Effusion," *Allergol Immunol* 15 (1987): 205–208.

30. D. S. Hurst, "Association of Otitis Media with Effusion and Allergy as Demonstrated by Intradermal Skin Testing and Eosinophil Protein Levels in Both Middle Ear Effusions and Mucosal Biopsies," *Laryngoscope* 106 (1996): 1128–1137.

31. G. I. Viscomi, "Allergic Secretory Otitis Media: An Approach to Management," *Laryngoscope* 85 (1975): 751–758.

32. T. M. Nsouli, S. M. Nsouli, R. E. Linde, et al., "Role of Food Allergy in Serious Otitis Media," *Ann Allergy* 73 (1994): 215–219.

33. E. M. Sarrell, H. A. Cohen, and E. Kahan, "Naturopathic Treatment for Ear Pain in Children," *Pediatrics* 111 (2003): 574–579.

34. J. H. Bland and S. M. Cooper, "Osteoarthritis: A Review of the Cell Biology Involved and Evidence for Reversibility: Management Rationally Related to Known Genesis and Pathophysiology," *Semin Arthritis Rheum* 14 (1984): 106–133.

35. G. H. Perry, M. J. Smith, and C. G. Whiteside, "Spontaneous Recovery of the Hip Joint Space in Degenerative Hip Disease," *Ann Rheum Dis* 31 (1972): 440–448.

36. J. B. Moseley, K. O'Malley, N. J. Petersen, et al., "A Controlled Trial of Arthroscopic Surgery for Osteoarthritis of the Knee. *N Engl J Med* 347(11) (2002): 81–8.

37. M. J. Shield, "Anti-Inflammatory Drugs and Their Effects on Cartilage Synthesis and Renal Function," *Eur J Rheumatol Inflam* 13 (1993): 7–16.

38. P. M. Brooks, S. R. Potter, and W. W. Buchanan, "NSAID and Osteoarthritis—Help or Hindrance," *J Rheumatol* 9 (1982): 3–5.

39. N. M. Newman and R. S. Ling, "Acetabular Bone Destruction Related to Non-Steroidal Anti-Inflammatory Drugs," *Lancet* 2 (1985): 11–13.

40. L. Solomon, "Drug Induced Arthropathy and Necrosis of the Femoral Head," *J Bone Joint Surg* 55 (1973): 246–261.

41. H. Ronningen and N. Langeland, "Indomethacin Treatment in Osteoarthritis of the Hip Joint," *Acta Orthop Scand* 50 (1979): 169–174.

42. J. Y. Reginster, O. Bruyere, and A. Neuprez, "Current Role of Glucosamine in the Treatment of Osteoarthritis," *Rheumatology* 46(5) (2007): 731–735.

43. T. E. Towheed, L. Maxwell, T. P. Anastassiades, et al., "Glucosamine Therapy for Treating Osteoarthritis," *Cochrane Database Syst Rev* 2 (2005): CD002946

44. J. W. Anderson, R. J. Nicolosi, and J. F. Borzelleca, "Glucosamine Effects in Humans: A Review of Effects on Glucose Metabolism, Side Effects, Safety Considerations, and Efficacy," *Food Chem Toxicol* 2 (February 2005): 187–201.

6. Creating a Market versus Providing a Cure

1. J. E. Rossouw, G. L. Anderson, R. L. Prentice, et al., "Risks and Benefits of Estrogen Plus Progestin in Healthy Postmenopausal Women: Principal Results from the Women's Health Initiative Randomized Controlled Trial," *JAMA* 288 (2002): 321–333.

2. S. Hulley, D. Grady, T. Bush, et al., "Randomized Trial of Estrogen Plus Progestin for Secondary Prevention of Coronary Heart Disease in Postmenopausal Women, Heart and Estrogen/Progestin Replacement Study (HERS) Research Group," *JAMA* 208 (1998): 605–613.

3. S. R. Heckbert, N. S. Weiss, T. D. Koepsell, et al., "Duration of Estrogen Replacement Therapy in Relation to the Risk of Incident Myocardial Infarction in Postmenopausal Women," *Arch Intern Med* 157 (1997): 1330–1336.

4. F. Grodstein, J. E. Manson, and M. J. Stampfer, "Postmenopausal Hormone Use and Secondary Prevention of Coronary Events in the Nurses' Health Study: A Prospective, Observational Study," *Ann Intern Med* 135 (2001): 1–8.

5. D. Grady, D. Herrington, V. Bittner, et al., "Cardiovascular Disease Outcomes during 6.8 Years of Hormone Therapy: Heart and Estrogen/Progestin Replacement Study Follow-Up (HERS II)," *JAMA* 288 (2002): 49–57.

6. G. A. Colditz and B. Rosner, "Cumulative Risk of Breast Cancer to Age 70 Years According to Risk Factor Status: Data from the Nurses' Health Study," *Am J Epidemiol* 152 (2000): 950–964.

7. D. A. Berry and P. M. Ravdin, "Breast Cancer Trends: A Marriage between Clinical Trial Evidence and Epidemiology," *J Natl Cancer Inst* 99(15) (2007): 1139–1141.

8. M. Hammar, G. Berg, and R. Lindgren, "Does Physical Exercise Influence the Frequency of Postmenopausal Hot Flushes?" *Acta Obstet Gynecol Scand* 69 (1990): 409–412.

9. F. S. Dalais, G. E. Rice, M. L. Wahlqvist, et al. "Effects of Dietary Phytoestrogens in Postmenopausal Women," *Climacteric* 1(2) (1998): 124–129.

10. A. Brzezinski, H. Adlercreutz, R. Shaoul, et al., "Short-Term Effects of Phytoestrogen-Rich Diet on Postmenopausal Women," *Menopause* 4 (1997): 89–94.

11. P. Albertazzi, F. Pansini, M. Bottazzi, et al., "Dietary Soy Supplementation and Phytoestrogen Levels," *Obstet Gynecol* 94(2) (1999): 299–231.

12. P. Albertazzi, F. Pansini, G. Bonaccorsi, et al., "The Effect of Dietary Soy Supplementation on Hot Flushes," *Obstet Gynecol* 91 (1998): 6–11.

13. M. Messina, and C. Hughes, "Efficacy of Soyfoods and Soybean Isoflavone Supplements for Alleviating Menopausal Symptoms Is Positively Related to Initial Hot Flush Frequency," *J Med Food* 6(1) (2003): 1–11.

14. D. H. Upmalis, R. Lobo, L. Bradley, et al., "Vasomotor Symptom Relief by Soy Isoflavone Extract Tablets in Postmenopausal Women: A Multicenter, Double-Blind, Randomized, Placebo-Controlled Study," *Menopause* 7 (2000): 236–242.

15. C. J. Haggans, A. M. Hutchins, B. A. Olson, et al., "Effect of Flaxseed Consumption on Urinary Estrogen Metabolites in Postmenopausal Women," *Nutr Cancer* 33(2) (1999): 188–195.

16. C. J. Haggans, E. J. Travelli, W. Thomas, et al., "The Effect of Flaxseed and Wheat Bran Consumption on Urinary Estrogen Metabolites in Premenopausal Women," *Cancer Epidemiol Biomarkers Prev* 9(7) (2000): 719–725.

17. W. Stoll, "Phytopharmacon Influences Atrophic Vaginal Epithelium: Double-Blind Study—*Cimicifuga* versus Estrogenic Substances," *Therapeuticum* 1 (1987): 23–31.

18. R. E. Nappi, B. Malavasi, B. Brundu, and F. Facchinetti, "Efficacy of *Cimicifuga racemosa* on Climacteric Complaints: A Randomized Study versus Low-Dose Transdermal Estradiol," *Gynecol Endocrinol* 20(1) (2005): 30–35.

19. R. Osmers, M. Friede, E. Liske, et al., "Efficacy and Safety of Isopropanolic Black Cohosh Extract for Climacteric Symptoms," *Obstet Gynecol* 105(5, Part 1) (2005): 1074–1083.

20. J. X. Li and Z. Y. Yu, "*Cimicifugae rhizoma*: From Origins, Bioactive Constituents to Clinical Outcomes," *Curr Med Chem* 13(24) (2006): 2927–2951.

21. L. A. Hidalgo, P. A. Chedraui, N. Morocho, et al., "The Effect of Red Clover Isoflavones on Menopausal Symptoms, Lipids, and Vaginal Cytology in Menopausal Women: A Randomized, Double-blind, Placebo-controlled Study," *Gynecol Endocrinol* 21(5) (2005): 257–264.

22. P. H. Linksvan de Weijer and R. Barentsen, "Isoflavones from Red Clover (Promensil) Significantly Reduce Menopausal Hot Flush Symptoms Compared with Placebo," *Maturitas* 42(3) (2002): 187–193.

23. S. C. Schuit, M. van der Klift, A. E. Weel, et al. "Fracture Incidence and Association with Bone Mineral Density in Elderly Men and Women: The Rotterdam Study," *Bone* 34(1) (2004): 195–202

24. J. Robbins, A. K. Aragaki, C. Kooperberg, et al., "Factors Associated with 5-Year Risk of Hip Fracture in Postmenopausal Women," *JAMA* 298(20) (2007): 2389–2398.

25. M. Sinaki, "Falls, Fractures, and Hip Pads," *Curr Osteoporos Rep* 2(4) (2004): 131–137.

26. D. M. Black, S. R. Cummings, D. B. Karpf, et al., "Randomised Trial of Effect of Alendronate on Risk of Fracture in Women with Existing Vertebral Fractures, Fracture Intervention Trial Research Group," *Lancet* 348(9041) (1996): 1535–1541.

27. M. Stevenson, M. L. Jones, E. De Nigris, et al., "A Systematic Review and Economic Evaluation of Alendronate, Etidronate, Risedronate, Raloxifene, and Teriparatide for the Prevention and Treatment of Postmenopausal Osteoporosis," *Health Technol Assess* 9(22) (2005): 1–160.

28. K. T. Borer, "Physical Activity in the Prevention and Amelioration of Osteoporosis in Women: Interaction of Mechanical, Hormonal, and Dietary Factors," *Sports Med* 35(9) 2005: 779–830.

29. C. M. Francucci, S. Rilli, P. Fiscaletti, and M. Boscaro, "Role of Vitamin K on Biochemical Markers, Bone Mineral Density, and Fracture Risk," *J Endocrinol Invest* 30(Suppl. 6) (2007): 24–28.

30. A. M. Smith, "Veganism and Osteoporosis: A Review of the Current Literature," *Int J Nurs Pract* 12(5) (2006): 302–306.

31. K. L. Tucker, K. Morita, N. Qiao, et al., "Colas, but Not Other Carbonated Beverages, Are Associated with Low Bone Mineral Density in Older Women: The Framingham Osteoporosis Study," *Am J Clin Nutr* 84(4) (2006): 936–942.

32. J. A. Thom, J. E. Morris, A. Bishop, and N. J. Blacklock, "The Influence of Refined Carbohydrate on Urinary Calcium Excretion," *Br J Urol* 50 (1978): 459–464.

33. R. P. Heaney, "Role of Dietary Sodium in Osteoporosis," *J Am Coll Nutr* 25(Suppl. 3) (June 2006): 271S–276S.

34. G. Isaia, P. D'Amelio, S. Di Bella, and C. Tamone, "Protein Intake: The Impact on Calcium and Bone Homeostasis," *J Endocrinol Invest* 30(Suppl. 6) (2007): 48–53.

35. M. Messina, S. Ho, and D. L. Alekel, "Skeletal Benefits of Soy Isoflavones: A Review of the Clinical Trial and Epidemiologic Data," *Curr Opin Clin Nutr Metab Care* 7(6) (2004): 649–658.

36. K. M. Newton, A. Z. LaCroix, L. Levy, et al., "Soy Protein and Bone Mineral Density in Older Men and Women: A Randomized Trial," *Maturitas* 55(3) (2006): 270–277.

37. D. Feskanich, W. C. Willett, M. J. Stampfer, and G. A. Colditz, "Milk, Dietary Calcium, and Bone Fractures in Women: A 12-Year Prospective Study," *Am J Public Health* 87(6) (1997): 992–997.

38. L. Xu, P. McElduff, C. D'Este, and J. Attia, "Does Dietary Calcium Have a Protective Effect on Bone Fractures in Women? A Meta-Analysis of Observational Studies," *Br J Nutr* 91 (2004): 625–634.

39. R. Rizzoli, S. Boonen, M. L. Brandi, et al., "The Role of Calcium and Vitamin D in the Management of Osteoporosis," *Bone* 42(2) (2008): 246–249.

40. S. Boonen, D. Vanderschueren, P. Haentjens, and P. Lips, "Calcium and Vitamin D in the Prevention and Treatment of Osteoporosis—A Clinical Update," *J Intern Med* 259(6) (2006): 539–552.

41. M. F. Holick, "The Role of Vitamin D for Bone Health and Fracture Prevention," *Curr Osteoporos Rep* 4(3) (September 2006): 96–102.

42. H. A. Bischoff-Ferrari, W. C. Willett, et al., "Fracture Prevention with Vitamin D Supplementation: A Meta-Analysis of Randomized Controlled Trials," *JAMA* 293(18) (2005): 2257–2264.

43. R. K. Rude and H. E. Gruber, "Magnesium Deficiency and Osteoporosis: Animal and Human Observations," *J Nutr Biochem* 15(12) (December 2004): 710–716.

44. B. Kitchin and S. L. Morgan, "Not Just Calcium and Vitamin D: Other Nutritional Considerations in Osteoporosis," *Curr Rheumatol Rep* 9(1) (2007): 85–92.

45. R. R. McLean and M. T. Hannan, "B Vitamins, Homocysteine, and Bone Disease: Epidemiology and Pathophysiology," *Curr Osteoporos Rep* 5(3) (2007): 112–119.

46. C. Palacios, "The Role of Nutrients in Bone Health, from A to Z," *Crit Rev Food Sci Nutr* 46(8) (2006): 621–628.

47. J. Iwamoto, T. Takeda, and Y. Sato, "Menatetrenone (Vitamin K_2 and Bone Quality in the Treatment of Postmenopausal Osteoporosis," *Nutr Rev* 64(12) (2006): 509–517.

48. M. H. Knapen, L. J. Schurgers, and C. Vermeer, "Vitamin K_2 Supplementation Improves Hip Bone Geometry and Bone Strength Indices in Postmenopausal Women," *Osteoporos Int* 18(7) (2007): 963–972. Review.

49. P. Autier and S. Gandini, "Vitamin D Supplementation and Total Mortality: A Meta-Analysis of Randomized Controlled Trials," *Arch Intern Med* 167(16) (2007): 1730–1737.

50. M. F. Holick, "The Vitamin D Epidemic and Its Health Consequences," *J Nutr* 135(11) (2005): 2739S–2748S.

51. J. B. Richards, A. M. Valdes, J. P. Gardner, et al., "Higher Serum Vitamin D Concentrations Are Associated with Longer Leukocyte Telomere Length in Women," *Am J Clin Nutr* 86(5) (2007): 1420–1425.

52. T. C. Chen, F. Chimeh, Z. Lu, et al., "Factors That Influence the Cutaneous Synthesis and Dietary Sources of Vitamin D," *Arch Biochem Biophys* 460(2) (2007): 213–217.

53. M. F. Holick, "Optimal Vitamin D Status for the Prevention and Treatment of Osteoporosis," *Drugs Aging* 24(12) (2007): 1017–1029.

7. Exploiting the Cholesterol Myth

1. Heart Protection Study Collaborative Group, "MRC: BHF Heart Protection Study of Cholesterol Lowering with Simvastatin in 20,536 High-Risk Individuals: A Randomised Placebo-Controlled Trial," *Lancet* 360 (2002): 7–22.

2. P. Thavendiranathan, A. Bagai, M. A. Brookhart, and N. K. Choudhry, "Primary Prevention of Cardiovascular Diseases with Statin Therapy: A meta-Analysis of Randomized Controlled Trials," *Arch Intern Med* 166(21) (November 2006): 2307–2313.

3. Cholesterol Treatment Trialists' (CTT) Collaborators, "Efficacy and Safety of Cholesterol-Lowering Treatment: Prospective Meta-Analysis of Data from 90,056 Participants in 14 Randomised Trials of Statins," *Lancet* 366 (2005): 1267–1278.

4. M. Vrecer, S. Turk, J. Drinovec, and A. Mrhar, "Use of Statins in Primary and Secondary Prevention of Coronary Heart Disease and Ischemic Stroke: Meta-Analysis of Randomized Trials," *Int J Clin Pharmacol Ther* 41(12) (2003): 567–577.

5. A. A. Hakim, H. Petrovitch, C. M. Burchfiel, et al., "Effects of Walking on Mortality among Nonsmoking Retired Men," *N Engl J Med* 338(2) (1998): 94–99.

6. A. Naska, E. Oikonomou, A. Trichopoulou, et al., "Siesta in Healthy Adults and Coronary Mortality in the General Population," *Arch Intern Med* 167(3) (2007): 296–301.

7. G. P. Littarru and P. Langsjoen, "Coenzyme Q10 and Statins: Biochemical and Clinical Implications," *Mitochondrion* 7(Suppl.) (2007): S168–S174.

8. J. Abramson and J. Wright, "Are Lipid-Lowering Guidelines Evidence-Based?" *Lancet* 369 (2007): 168–169.

9. J. M. E. Walsh and M. Pigame, "Drug Treatment of Hyperlipidemia in Women," *JAMA* 291 (2004): 2243–2252.

10. J. Shepherd, G. J. Blauw, M. B. Murphy, et al., "Pravastatin in Elderly Individuals at Risk of Vascular Disease (PROSPER): A randomised Controlled Trial," *Lancet* 360 (2002): 1623–1630.

11. ALLHAT Officers and Coordinators for ALLHAT Collaborative Research
     Group, Antihypertensive and Lipid-Lowering Treatment to Prevent Heart
     Attack Trial, "Major Outcomes in Moderately Hypercholesterolemic,
     Hypertensive Patients Randomized to Pravastatin versus Usual Care," *JAMA*
     288(23): 2998–3007.

12. N. Nakaya, T. Kita, H. Mabuchi, et al., "Large-Scale Cohort Study on
     the Relationship between Serum Lipid Concentrations and Risk of
     Cerebrovascular Disease under Low-Dose Simvastatin in Japanese Patients
     with Hypercholesterolemia: Sub-Analysis of the Japan Lipid Intervention
     Trial (J-LIT)," *Circ J* 69(9) (2005): 1016–1021.

13. H. S. Hecht and S. M. Harman, "Relation of Aggressiveness of Lipid-
     Lowering Treatment to Changes in Calcified Plaque Burden by Electron
     Beam Tomography," *Am J Cardiol* 92(3) (2003): 334–336.

14. D. J. Jenkins, C. W. Kendall, A. Marchie, et al., "Effects of a Dietary Portfolio
     of Cholesterol-Lowering Foods versus Lovastatin on Serum Lipids and
     C-Reactive Protein," *JAMA* 290 (2003): 502–510.

15. M. De Lorgeril, P. Salen, J.-L. Martin, et al., "Mediterranean Diet, Traditional
     Risk Factors, and the Rate of Cardiovascular Complications after Myocardial
     Infarction: Final Report of the Lyon Diet Heart Study," *Circulation* 99 (1999):
     779–785.

16. L. Serra-Majem, B. Roman, and R. Estruch, "Scientific Evidence of
     Interventions Using the Mediterranean Diet: A systematic Review," *Nutr Rev*
     64(2, Part 2) (2006): S27–S47.

17. K. Esposito, R. Marfella, M. Ciotola, et al., "Effect of a Mediterranean-Style
     Diet on Endothelial Dysfunction and Markers of Vascular Inflammation in
     the Metabolic Syndrome: A Randomized Trial," *JAMA* 292(12) (2004): 1440–
     1446.

18. J. R. Guyton, "Niacin in Cardiovascular Prevention: Mechanisms, Efficacy,
     and Safety," *Curr Opin Lipidol* 18(4) (2007): 415–420.

19. P. L. Canner, K. G. Berge, and N. K. Wenger, "Fifteen-Year Mortality in
     Coronary Drug Project Patients: Long-Term Benefit with Niacin," *J Am Coll
     Cardiol* 8 (1986): 1245–1255.

20. D. R. Illingworth, E. A. Stein, Y. B. Mitchel, et al., "Comparative Effects of
     Lovastatin and Niacin in Primary Hypercholesterolemia," *Arch Intern Med* 14
     (1994): 1586–1595.

21. J. T. Van, J. Pan, T. Wasty, et al., "Comparison of Extended-Release Niacin and Atorvastatin Monotherapies and Combination Treatment of the Atherogenic Lipid Profile in Diabetes Mellitus," *Am J Cardiol* 89 (2002): 1306–1308.

22. S. M. Grundy, G. L. Vega, M. E. McGovern, et al., "Efficacy, Safety, and Tolerability of Once-Daily Niacin for the Treatment of Dyslipidemia Associated with Type 2 Diabetes: Results of the Assessment of Diabetes Control and Evaluation of the Efficacy of Niaspan Trial," *Arch Intern Med* 162 (2002): 1568–1576.

23. J. R. Guyton and H. E. Bays, "Safety Considerations with Niacin Therapy," *Am J Cardiol* 99(6A) (2007): 22C–31C.

24. B. G. Brown, X.-Q. Zhao, A. Chait, et al., "Simvastatin and Niacin, Antioxidant Vitamins, or the Combination for the Prevention of Coronary Disease," *N Engl J Med* 345 (2001): 1583–1592.

25. J. M. Roza, Z. Xian-Liu, and N. Guthrie, "Effect of Citrus Flavonoids and Tocotrienols on Serum Cholesterol Levels in Hypercholesterolemic Subjects," *Altern Ther Health Med* 13(6) (2007): 44–48.

26. T. A. Jacobson, "Beyond Lipids: The Role of Omega-3 Fatty Acids from Fish Oil in the Prevention of Coronary Heart Disease," *Curr Atheroscler Rep* 9(2) (2007): 145–153.

27. C. Wang, W. S. Harris, M. Chung, et al., "N-3 Fatty Acids from Fish or Fish-Oil Supplements, but Not Alpha-Linolenic Acid, Benefit Cardiovascular Disease Outcomes in Primary- and Secondary-Prevention Studies: A Systematic Review," *Am J Clin Nutr* 84(1) (July 2006): 5–17.

28. C. von Schacky and W. S. Harris, "Cardiovascular Risk and the Omega-3 Index," *J Cardiovasc Med* 8(Suppl. 1) (2007): S46–S49.

29. C. H. Ruxton, S. C. Reed, M. J. Simpson, and K. J. Millington, "The Health Benefits of Omega-3 Polyunsaturated Fatty Acids: A Review of the Evidence," *J Hum Nutr Diet* 20(3) (2007): 275–285.

30. C. von Schacky, "A Review of Omega-3 Ethyl Esters for Cardiovascular Prevention and Treatment of Increased Blood Triglyceride Levels," *Vasc Health Risk Manag* 2(3) (2006): 251–262.

31. A. Rozanski, J. A. Blumenthal, K. W. Davidson, et al., "The Epidemiology, Pathophysiology, and Management of Psychosocial Risk Factors in Cardiac Practice: The Emerging Field of Behavioral Cardiology," *J Am Coll Cardiol* 45(5) (2005): 637–651.

8. Drugs Are Less Powerful Than our Attitude

1. J. Moncrieff and I. Kirsch, "Efficacy of Antidepressants in Adults," *BMJ* 331 (2005): 155–157.

2. I. Kirsch, T. J. Moore, A. Scoboria, and S. S. Nicholls, "The Emperor's New Drugs: An Analysis of Antidepressant Medication Data Submitted to the U.S. Food and Drug Administration," *Prevention and Treatment* 5(1) (2002).

3. A. T. Beck, "The Current State of Cognitive Therapy: A 40-Year Retrospective," *Arch Gen Psychiatry* 62(9) (2005): 953–959.

4. J. D. Davis and G. Tremont, "Neuropsychiatric Aspects of Hypothyroidism and Treatment Reversibility," *Minerva Endocrinol* 32(1) (2007): 49–65.

5. K. Kreitsch, "Prevalence, Presenting Symptoms, and Psychological Characteristics of Individuals Experiencing a Diet-Related Mood Disturbance," *Behav Ther* 19 (1985): 593–594.

6. P. Salmon, "Effects of Physical Exercise on Anxiety, Depression, and Sensitivity to Stress: A Unifying Theory," *Clin Psychol Rev* 21(1) (2001): 33–61.

7. M. T. Murray, *5-HTP—The Natural Way to Overcome Depression, Obesity, and Insomnia* (New York: Bantam, 1998).

8. D. Healy, "Did Regulators Fail over Selective Serotonin Reuptake Inhibitors?" *BMJ* 333 (2006): 92–95.

9. D. Fergusson, S. Doucette, K. C. Glass, et al., "Association between Suicide Attempts and Selective Serotonin Reuptake Inhibitors: Systematic Review of Randomised Controlled Trials," *BMJ* 330(7488) (2005): 396. Review.

10. C. B. Nemeroff, A. Kalali, M. B. Keller, et al., "Impact of Publicity Concerning Pediatric Suicidality Data on Physician Practice Patterns in the United States," *Arch Gen Psychiatry* 64(4) (2007): 466–472.

11. T. L. Schwartz, N. Nihalani, S. Jindal, et al., "Psychiatric Medication-Induced Obesity: A Review." *Obes Rev* 5(2) (2004): 115–121.

12. M. B. Raeder, I. Bjelland, S. Emil Vollset, and V. M. Steen, "Obesity, Dyslipidemia, and Diabetes with Selective Serotonin Reuptake Inhibitors: The Hordaland Health Study," *J Clin Psychiatry* 67(12) (2006): 1974.

13. Hypericum Depression Trial Study Group, "Effect of *Hypericum perforatum* (St. John's Wort) in Major Depressive Disorder: A Randomized Controlled Trial," *JAMA* 287(14) (2002): 1807–1814.

14. M. Gastpar, A. Singer, and K. Zeller, "Efficacy and Tolerability of Hypericum Extract STW3 in Long-Term Treatment with a Once-Daily Dosage in Comparison with Sertraline," *Pharmacopsychiatry* 38(2) (2005): 78–86.

15. A. Szegedi, R. Kohnen, A. Dienel, and M. Kieser, "Acute Treatment of Moderate to Severe Depression with Hypericum Extract WS 5570 (St. John's Wort): Randomised Controlled Double Blind Non-Inferiority Trial versus Paroxetine," *BMJ* 330(7490) (2005): 503.

9. Drugs Cannot Overcome a Poor Diet or an Unhealthy Lifestyle

1. K. J. Duffey, P. Gordon-Larsen, D. R. Jacobs Jr., et al., "Differential Associations of Fast Food and Restaurant Food Consumption with 3-Y Change in Body Mass Index: The Coronary Artery Risk Development in Young Adults Study," *Am J Clin Nutr* 85(1) (2007): 201–208.

2. R. Sturm and K. B. Wells, "Does Obesity Contribute as Much to Morbidity as Poverty or Smoking?" *Public Health* 115 (2001): 229–295.

3. S. Bolen, L. Feldman, J. Vassy, et al., "Systematic Review: Comparative Effectiveness and Safety of Oral Medications for Type 2 Diabetes Mellitus," *Ann Intern Med* 147(6) (2007): 386–399.

4. H. Thisted, S. P. Johnsen, and J. Rungby, "Sulfonylureas and the Risk of Myocardial Infarction," *Metabolism* 55(Suppl. 1) (May 2006): S16–S19.

5. E. Mannucci, M. Monami, G. Masotti, and N. Marchionni, "All-Cause Mortality in Diabetic Patients Treated with Combinations of Sulfonylureas and Biguanides," *Diabetes Metab Res Rev* 20(1) (2004): 44–47.

6. S. E. Nissen and K. Wolski, "Effect of Rosiglitazone on the Risk of Myocardial Infarction and Death from Cardiovascular Causes," *N Engl J Med* 356(24) (2007): 2457–2471.

7.   W. C. Knowler, E. Barrett-Connor, S. E. Fowler, et al., "Reduction in the Incidence of Type 2 Diabetes with Lifestyle Intervention or Metformin," *N Engl J Med* 346(6) (2002): 393–403.

8.   R. Dhingra, L. Sullivan, P. F. Jacques, et al., "Soft Drink Consumption and Risk of Developing Cardiometabolic Risk Factors and the Metabolic Syndrome in Middle-Aged Adults in the Community," *Circulation* 116(5) (2007): 480–488.

9.   L. J. Appel, T. J. Moore, E. Obarzanek, et al., "A Clinical Trial of the Effects of Dietary Patterns on Blood Pressure, DASH Collaborative Research Group," *N Engl J Med* 336 (1997): 1117–1124.

10.   F. M. Sacks, L. P. Svetkey, W. M. Vollmer, et al., "Effects on Blood Pressure of Reduced Dietary Sodium and the Dietary Approaches to Stop Hypertension (DASH) Diet, DASH-Sodium Collaborative Research Group," *N Engl J Med* 344 (2001): 3–10.

11.   P. K. Whelton and J. He, "Potassium in Preventing and Treating High Blood Pressure," *Semin Nephrol* 19 (1999): 494–499.

12.   H. Fujita, R. Yasumoto, M. Hasegawa, and K. Ohshima, "Antihypertensive Activity of 'Katsuobushi Oligopeptide' in Hypertensive and Borderline Hypertensive Subjects," *Jpn Pharmacol Ther* 25 (1997): 147–151.

13.   C. D. Boethel, "Sleep and the Endocrine System: New Associations to Old Diseases," *Curr Opin Pulm Med* 8 (2002): 502–505.

14.   J. E. Gangwisch, D. Malaspina, B. Boden-Albala, and S. B. Heymsfield, "Inadequate Sleep as a Risk Factor for Obesity: Analyses of the NHANES I," *Sleep* 28(10) (October 1, 2005): 1289–1296.

15.   J. E. Gangwisch, S. B. Heymsfield, B. Boden-Albala, et al., "Sleep Duration as a Risk Factor for Diabetes Incidence in a Large U.S. Sample," *Sleep* 30(12) (2007): 1667–1673.

16.   J. E. Gangwisch, S. B. Heymsfield, B. Boden-Albala, et al. "Short Sleep Duration as a Risk Factor for Hypertension: Analyses of the First National Health and Nutrition Examination Survey," *Hypertension* 47(5) (2006): 833–839.

17.   W. K. Al-Delaimy, J. E. Manson, W. C. Willett, et al., "Snoring as a Risk Factor for Type 2 Diabetes Mellitus: A Prospective Study," *Am J Epidemiol* 155 (2002): 387–393.

18. D. Pevernagie, E. Hamans, P. Van Cauwenberge, and R. Pauwels, "Related External Nasal Dilation Reduces Snoring in Chronic Rhinitis Patients: A Randomized Controlled Trial," *Eur Respir J* 15 (2000): 996–1000.

19. J. P. Kirkness, J. R. Wheatley, and T. C. Amis, "Nasal Airflow Dynamics: Mechanisms and Responses Associated with an External Nasal Dilator Strip," *Eur Respir J* 15 (2000): 929–936.

20. S. Taheri, L. Lin, D. Austin, et al., "Short Sleep Duration Is Associated with Reduced Leptin, Elevated Ghrelin, and Increased Body Mass Index," *Public Library Science Med* 1(3) (2004): e62.

10. Looking behind the Headlines and through the Bias

1. S. Bent, C. Kane, K. Shinohara, et al., "Saw Palmetto for Benign Prostatic Hyperplasia," *N Engl J Med* 354(6) (2006): 557–566.

2. T. Wilt, A. Ishani, and R. MacDonald, "*Serenoa repens* for Benign Prostatic Hyperplasia," *Cochrane Database Syst Rev* 3 (2002): CD001423.

3. P. Boyle, C. Robertson, F. Lowe, and C. Roehrborn, "Updated Meta-Analysis of Clinical Trials of *Serenoa repens* Extract in the Treatment of Symptomatic Benign Prostatic Hyperplasia," *BJU Int* 93(6) (2004): 751–756.

4. L. Hooper, R. L. Thompson, R. A. Harrison, et al., "Risks and Benefits of Omega-3 Fats for Mortality, Cardiovascular Disease, and Cancer: Systematic Review," *BMJ* 332 (2006): 752–760.

5. L. Hooper, R. Riemersma, P. Durrington, et al., "Authors' reply–Omega-3s and Health," BMJ.com (April 7, 2006).

6. "Effects of Omega-3 Fatty Acids on Cardiovascular Disease," http://www.ahcpr.gov/clinic/epcsums/o3cardsum.htm/dec.2004

7. C. M. Albert, H. Campos, M. J. Stampfer, et al., "Blood Levels of Long-Chain n-3 Fatty Acids and the Risk of Sudden Death," *N Engl J Med* 346(15) (2002): 1113–1118.

8. E. Guallar, M. I. Sanz-Gallardo, P. van't Veer, et al., "Mercury, Fish Oils, and the Risk of Myocardial Infarction," *N Engl J Med* 347 (2002): 1747–1754.

9. J. Lazarou, B. H. Pomeranz, and P. N. Corey, "Incidence of Adverse Drug Reactions in Hospitalized Patients: A Meta-Analysis of Prospective Studies," *JAMA* 279(15) (1998): 1200–1205.

10. L. A. Thomsen, A. G. Winterstein, B. Søndergaard, et al., "Systematic Review of the Incidence and Characteristics of Preventable Adverse Drug Events in Ambulatory Care," *Ann Pharmacother.* 41(9) (2007): 1411–1426.

11. L. Hazell and S. A. Shakir, "Under-Reporting of Adverse Drug Reactions: A Systematic Review," *Drug Saf* 29(5) (2006): 385–396.

12. J. S. Goodwin and M. R. Tangum, "Battling Quackery: Attitudes about Micronutrient Supplements in American Academic Medicine," *Arch Intern Med* 158(20) (1998): 2187–2191.

13. G. P. Oakley, "Folic Acid—Preventable Spina Bifida and Anencephaly," *JAMA* 269 (1993): 1292–1293.

14. S. Bo and E. Pisu, "Role of Dietary Magnesium in Cardiovascular Disease Prevention, Insulin Sensitivity, and Diabetes," *Curr Opin Lipidol* 19(1) (2008): 50–56.

15. M. Barbagallo and L. J. Dominguez, "Magnesium Metabolism in Type 2 Diabetes Mellitus, Metabolic Syndrome, and Insulin Resistance," *Arch Biochem Biophys* 458(1) (2007): 40–47.

16. Y. Song, K. He, E. B. Levitan, et al., "Effects of Oral Magnesium Supplementation on Glycaemic Control in Type 2 Diabetes: A Meta-Analysis of Randomized Double-Blind Controlled Trials," *Diabet Med* 23(10) (2006): 1050–1056.

11. How to Get Well

1. T. Maruta, R. C. Colligan, M. Malinchoc, and K. P. Offord, "Optimism-Pessimism Assessed in the 1960s and Self-Reported Health Status 30 Years Later," *Mayo Clin Proc* 77(8) (2002): 748–753.

2. R. De Vogli, T. Chandola, and M. G. Marmot, "Negative Aspects of Close Relationships and Heart Disease," *Arch Intern Med* 167(18) (2007): 1951–1957.

INDEX